YOGA
SHALOM

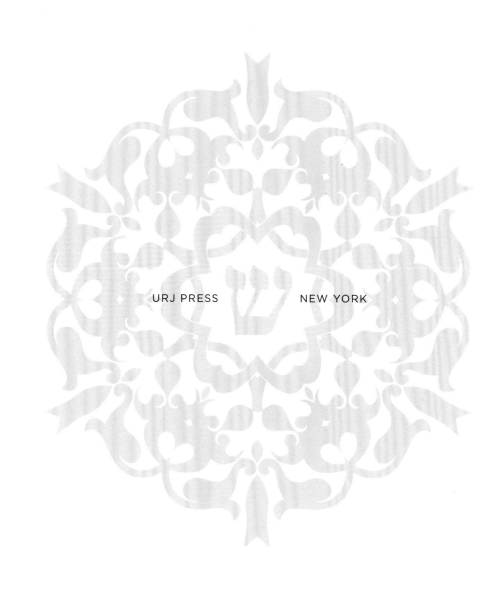

URJ PRESS   NEW YORK

YOGA SHALOM

LISA LEVINE *with* CAROL KRUCOFF

The material contained in *Yoga Shalom* is for educational purposes only.

Please consult your health care provider before beginning this program or any new physical activity. It is important to recognize that yoga involves some physical exertion and stretching, and it is each individual's responsibility to not exceed his or her limits in the practice of yoga. Be aware that not all postures or practices are suitable for everyone. **If any movement seems inappropriate for your body or causes discomfort or pain—please DO NOT DO IT!**

URJ Press disclaims all liability for any discomfort, loss, or injury connected with the practices presented in *Yoga Shalom*.

Library of Congress Cataloging-in-Publication Data

Levine, Lisa, 1959-
  Yoga shalom / Lisa Levine with Carol Krucoff.
    p. cm.
  ISBN 978-0-8074-1145-2
  1. Judaism--Liturgy. 2. Prayer--Judaism. 3. Yoga--Judaism. 4. Spiritual
life--Judaism. I. Krucoff, Carol. II. Title.
  BM660.L45 2012
  296.4'5--dc23
                        2011035207

URJ Press
633 Third Avenue
New York, NY 10017-6778
(212) 650-4120
Press@urj.org

This book is printed on acid-free paper.
Copyright © 2012 by URJ Press
Manufactured in the United States of America
10 9 8 7 6 5 4 3 2 1

CONTENTS

Part I: Introductory Prayers

Part II: The *Sh'ma* and Its Blessings

Part III: *Amidah*

Part IV: Concluding Prayers

YOGA
SHALOM

PREFACES

How does one embody prayer? This is a question I've been struggling with for more than twenty-five years, as both a practicing cantor and yoga practitioner. My journey began while I was studying at Hebrew Union College–Jewish Institute of Religion in New York, commuting from Brooklyn by subway, working

two student pulpits, studying voice, striving to achieve the highest level of success in my classes, and trying to remain functional in all of these areas. Stress was my constant companion. Yoga became the avenue I used to free my voice, reduce my stress, and focus my mind on the task at hand—namely, learning the art of the cantor. A crucial by-product: I learned to be more present in my prayers and meditations so I could better pray with and on the behalf of my congregation.

The next step on my journey came when I was asked to teach yoga at a cantors convention. I titled my class "Yoga for Singers." The very simple practice I taught enabled me to become a much better singer, not only with the expanded use of my lungs and diaphragm, but also in my capacity to open my chest and allow the free flow of air through my body.

My big breakthrough came along, though, when I was invited to lead a yoga worship service at the URJ Biennial Convention in Minneapolis in 1995. My partner on this maiden voyage was Rabbi Susie Moskowitz. She had done some work combining Jewish prayer and yoga, so she provided a framework for some of the prayers in our service. The more I thought about it, the more I began to connect certain yoga postures with certain prayers, like the Sun Salutation with *Yotzeir Or* and the forward bend with *Bar'chu.* I also created a CD so that I could participate fully in the service without doing live music.

After my initial experience with yoga worship, I began envisioning the prayers in all of my yoga classes and interpreting which asanas (yoga postures) would fit best with each prayer. It is through this process that I began to create my vision of the embodiment of the prayers of the *Shacharit* (morning) service.

It all came together rather quickly after that. When I went out as artist-in-residence to different communities, which I often did to share my liturgical musical compositions, I would teach yoga worship as part of my offerings. One community I visited was Judea Reform Congregation in Durham, North Carolina, and that Shabbat morning several yoga teachers were in attendance. One in particular, Carol Krucoff, took an interest in my yoga worship service. Carol was a journalist and author, who frequently contributed to *Yoga Journal*. She had some suggestions about the yoga postures offered, and as we talked, we became excited about the idea of writing a book together that might be beneficial to Jewish yoga practitioners everywhere. *Yoga Shalom* was born.

The resulting book is now before you. *Yoga Shalom* is first and foremost a Jewish worship service that follows a format that resembles a prayer book. The yoga postures and breathing practices that accompany the service are meant as a guide for understanding both the subtleties of Jewish worship as well as the ancient spiritual discipline of yoga.

What makes the practice of yoga so compatible with Jewish worship? I believe it is the shared history of a deep physical connection to prayer. As a people, we have always had certain physical choreographies that accompany our prayers, such as bowing during *Aleinu* or rising three times on our toes during the *K'dushah*. Yoga and Jewish worship share the goal of opening practioners to a deep connection with a higher power, and some contemporary modes of Jewish worship have incorporated prayers for healing and meditation as a tool for spirituality. Finally, our strong communal experience as a tribal people unites us together as we strive for wholeness and a fuller, more spiritual connection to ourselves, our congregations, and our world. Judaism and yoga are completely compatible in reaching these goals.

Embodying prayer is not as simple as practicing yoga. One must also understand the content of prayer, its context in history, and why each prayer was selected for its place in the worship service. Ultimately, the power of prayer comes from what each of us brings from our spirits. That is discovered through the deep exploration of breath, stillness of mind, and challenging of body. While my search continues for enlightenment and true embodiment of prayer, I know that I am deep into my journey, and I look forward to bringing others into the vast unknown of what has proved to be the greatest adventure of my lifetime: seeking Oneness through yoga, meditation, music, and prayer chant. It is a journey that will never end as I continue to discover the hidden godliness in myself and in others.

Namaste,
Lisa

Throughout my life, I've embraced physical activity as a powerful vehicle for connecting with the Divine. I've often felt closest to God while moving my body through space, feeling the precious gifts of breath in my lungs and energy in my limbs, supported by the grateful beating of my heart. I danced ballet during my early years and minored in dance in college. In my early twenties I started running and also began taking a weekly yoga class, both to enhance flexibility and to relieve stress. When my children were young, I studied martial arts with them, earning a second-degree black belt. Throughout my adult life, yoga has always been a refuge—a practice of turning within and connecting with my deepest self.

As a journalist, my writing has focused on the profound connection between physical activity and health, and I specialize in articles about "Movement as Medicine." From 1988 to 2000, I wrote a syndicated column on this topic for the *Washington Post*, called "Bodyworks," and compiled essential information into a book, *Healing Moves: How to Cure, Relieve and Prevent Common Ailments with Exercise*, coauthored with my cardiologist husband, Mitchell Krucoff, which was published in 2000. In our sedentary, computerized culture—where, sadly, most people are inactive—my goal is to encourage people to restore the joy of recess, to empower them to move their bodies to enhance health of mind, body, and spirit.

In 1999, I decided to train as a yoga teacher to deepen my own practice. I was in my mid-forties and recognized that, unlike karate, yoga was a practice I could continue for the rest of my life. During my teacher training I was required to do a service project and volunteered to teach yoga to older adult veterans at the Durham, North Carolina, Veterans Affairs Medical Center. The requirement was for twelve hours of community service, but I continued volunteering at the VA for five years, teaching a weekly yoga class for the Gerofit gerontology rehab program, because this experience was so rewarding. These older adult veterans were not your typical yoga students—in fact, many had little knowledge of yoga and kept teasing me about "what kind of yogurt" I'd be offering. Most had numerous health conditions including heart disease, arthritis, hypertension, and diabetes. Creating an appropriate yoga practice was challenging, but I discovered that even relatively gentle movement—combined with yogic breath and the practice's attitudes of compassion and "non-striving"—offered these students great benefit. They told me they slept better, their arthritis pain diminished, and some even reported improvements in their blood pressure. I was hooked on teaching yoga to people with health challenges and pursued further training in this area, becoming a yoga therapist at Duke Integrative Medicine in 2007.

When Lisa came to our synagogue to teach *Yoga Shalom*, I signed up with great interest, because the yoga practice has always been—for me—a form of prayer. I loved the experience she created, with beautiful music and heartfelt prayers accompanying the posture practice. I particularly enjoyed praying in Hebrew, because as a practice that originated in India, yoga is typically associated with chants in Sanskrit. Lisa had created an extraordinary opportunity for people to pray not just with their mouths and minds, but with their breath, bodies, and hearts.

It has been an honor and a pleasure to help create this unique worship service, and it is my sincere hope that practicing *Yoga Shalom* will offer people a new way to connect within, with each other, and with God.

L'Shalom,
Carol

INTRODUCTION

Yoga Shalom is a spiritual and physical journey, guided by a sequence of traditional Hebrew morning prayers. Although the weekday *Shacharit* service serves as the textual basis for *Yoga Shalom*, you can practice this worship service for body and soul at any time of day or on Shabbat. Before you begin,

prepare yourself and your environment. Give yourself at least one hour and fifteen minutes to devote to your spiritual, physical, and emotional well-being. Choose a space with plenty of room where you'll remain undisturbed. Turn off your cell phone and any other electronic distractions. You may enjoy lighting a candle and dimming the lights.

Yoga Shalom is for everyone, regardless of their level of yoga experience or physical abilities. *Yoga Shalom* will change your life by helping to relax your body, calm your mind, and nurture your spirit, while at the same time strengthening your body and enhancing your flexibility. You can practice *Yoga Shalom* at home, in a yoga studio, or at the synagogue, on a mat or in a chair.

Yoga Shalom is meant to be adaptable to your own needs, skills, and comfort level, so feel free to be creative and personalize your practice. You'll notice that there are advanced poses offered for each posture. You may wish to flow into these poses as you be-

come stronger and more accustomed to the content of the service. There are also modifications for less experienced practitioners and those with health challenges. As you become familiar with the soundtrack, chant along with the prayers and music. Consider keeping your own journal of writings, or personal *kavanot*, as you go.

The book is accompanied by a DVD and a CD. The CD includes original music written especially for *Yoga Shalom* as well as recordings from a number of talented Jewish artists. Music is an integral part of the *Yoga Shalom* experience, and each song has been carefully chosen to deepen the connection between body and spirit. The DVD guides you through the worship service and models the experience of leading it. When you feel comfortable enough with the service, you can then unplug from the video and begin to experience or lead the service with the book as your guide, listening and flowing through the yoga postures that embody each prayer.

Each prayer path contains the following:

+ The prayer in Hebrew with a creative translation into English

+ A narration that you will hear on the DVD or that you can read over the corresponding CD track

+ Directions for each yoga sequence, with options for deepening the practice

+ The yoga connection to each prayer path

+ The context of that path to Jewish prayer

+ A creative original *kavanah*, or creative interpretation, to give you an alternate window into the prayer

+ Questions for the prayer that challenge you to open your spirit to change

+ An area for you to write your own personal thoughts and intentions

We challenge you to create your own worship experience. This is your prayer, your practice, your time for yourself to devote to your well-being. Use this book as a guide, but never feel that it is meant to be static. Yoga is a journey, and worship is a journey, and we want to feel as though we are continually growing and challenging ourselves through that journey toward wholeness, strength, flexibility, and inner peace.

Yoga Shalom has the power to bring together—in a Jewish context—body, mind, and spirit. It is our hope that it can also be a catalyst for change. Worshiping outside the box of a traditional prayer service can even engage and unite your synagogue's professional staff, lay leadership, and members of your community, encouraging them to connect to their inner spirits and facilitate deeper connections with one another.

Most importantly, it can change your daily view of yourself, the world, and how you connect to it.

It is our prayer that you will want to experience the extraordinary benefits of *Yoga Shalom* again and again, in what we hope will lead you on your own path to self-awareness, understanding, acceptance, wholeness, and contentment in your own life's journey.

PART I

Introductory Prayers

INTRODUCTION: *Modeh/Modah Ani* ✦ MUSIC: "Flute Stream" by Ira Fein

מוֹדֶה / מוֹדָה אֲנִי לְפָנֶיךָ

Modeh/modah ani l' fanecha.

I am listening to my body. I am ready for prayer.

The first prayer of the section of prayers called *Birchot HaShachar*, the Morning Blessings, is *Modah Ani* (for a woman) / *Modeh Ani* (for a man). The first line literally means "I offer thanks to You, Holy One of Blessing, for restoring my soul to my body." We begin our preparation for worship with this prayer in gratitude for the gift of life and the acknowledgment of a higher power in the universe.

Come to a sitting position, *close your eyes, and begin to separate yourself from what has come before and what will come after this quiet time of renewal devoted to yourself and your well-being. This is your time to ready yourself for prayer. Imagine you are packing a suitcase with things in your life that are dragging you down, causing you stress, or making you unhappy. Put that suitcase outside the door. It will be waiting for you should you wish to take it with you after your practice, or you may choose to simply abandon it. Listen to your body today. Let go of any feelings of competition or self-judgment, and approach your practice with a sense of self-compassion and self-discovery. Attempt to be fully present and hear what your body and your spirit are telling you. If unwanted thoughts or "to do" lists pop into your mind, use your breath to release them and come back into the present moment.*

DIRECTIONS

Come to a comfortable sitting position on your mat or in a chair. Allow your sit bones, the bones at the base of your pelvis that support you when you're seated, to release down toward the earth, and extend the crown of your head up toward the heavens. Release any distracting thoughts, and turn your attention to your breath. Spend a few moments bringing your body and mind into stillness.

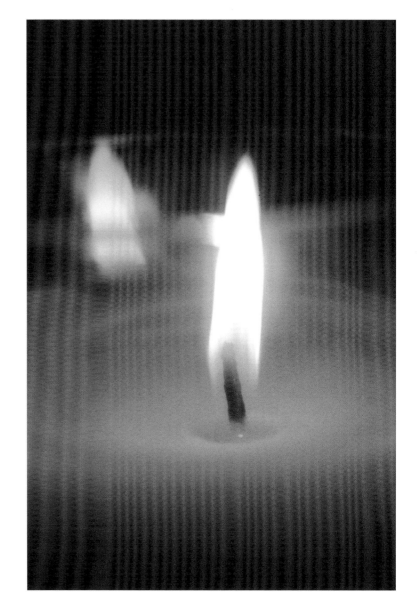

YOGA CONNECTION: UNION

Yoga is a profound spiritual discipline that originated more than five thousand years ago in India. The word "yoga" comes from the ancient Sanskrit word *yuj*, which means "to yoke" or "to unite." At the most basic level, yoga helps unite the body and mind. At a deeper level, yoga seeks to unite the individual with the Divine.

QUESTION

Is there an area of your mind you wish to quiet? Picture your thoughts floating away like clouds.

KAVANAH

I pray for peace of mind
For time to devote to myself
To release and let go
To separate from daily strivings.
I am ready, open to change
Connected yet disconnected
Fill me, O God, with the healing
Of your spirit.

PERSONAL KAVANAH

_____

_____

_____

1

בָּרוּךְ אַתָּה יְיָ, רוֹפֵא כָל בָּשָׂר וּמַפְלִיא לַעֲשׂוֹת.

Baruch atah Adonai, rofei chol basar umafli laasot.

Blessed are You, Holy One of Blessing, Healer of souls and Giver of strength.

We begin our journey with the prayer *Asher Yatzar*, the sixth prayer in the series of prayers called *Birchot HaShachar*, the Morning Blessings, which are an introductory series of offerings preparing us for the next section of the service. This prayer praises the Holy One for forming our bodies with skill and creating openings and closings crucial to our existence. Were one of these vital openings to fail, we would be unable to live. The *chatimah*, or very end of the prayer, is our guide: "Blessed are You, Holy One of Blessing, Healer of flesh and Worker of wonders."

Our mat today *is our* mishkan, *our holy place. In Hebrew, the word* n'shamah *means "soul." The word* n'shimah *means "breath." Our breath is linked to our soul. Through the practice of slowing and deepening our breath, we begin to open a place within our body that is symbolic of opening a pathway to God. We inhale through our nostrils and become aware of the many openings and organs that depend on the air that we breathe. We exhale through our nostrils, bringing cleansing warmth and energy into our body and releasing negative thoughts and stress. With each full inhalation, we deepen the connection to our spirituality and begin to unlock the emotions and thoughts hidden deep inside. Each exhalation connects our life force with that of the planet and creates an awareness of our connection to every living thing. As you deepen your breath and begin to release your emotions, feel them rising like bubbles in a stream, and allow them to flow through you and out into nature.*

DIRECTIONS

Continue to lengthen through the spine as you allow your eyelids to close. Rest your palms on your knees (*right*), or place the backs of your hands on your knees, touching your index finger to your thumb in the gesture known as *Gyan Mudra*, wherever your hands feel most comfortable. Or, if you're seated on the floor, feel free to bring your fingertips to your mat on either side of your body. Take full deep inhalations, inviting your breath to the low-

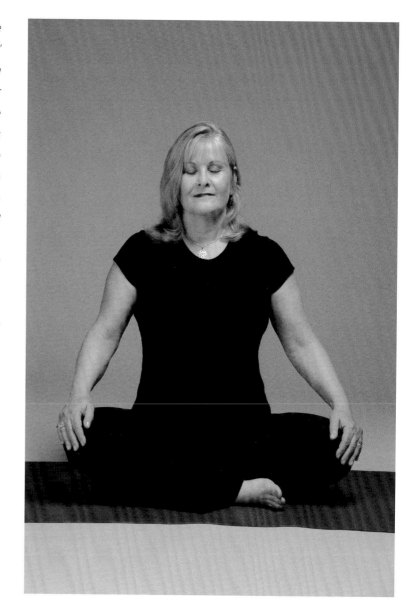

est part of the lungs so that you can feel your belly round, your rib cage expand out to the sides, and the space up under your collarbones broaden and fill. As you exhale, draw your navel to your spine and lift the crown of your head to the sky, chest proud and shoulders relaxed. With each inhalation, feel the expansion in your body as if you are filling a precious vessel. With each exhalation, release the old, used air as you also let go of unwanted stresses, concerns, and negative thoughts. While listening to the music, continue to ride the waves of your breath.

CHAIR MODIFICATION: *Sit tall in your chair, hands resting comfortably on your thighs or in your lap (appendix, fig. 1.1).*

ADVANCED TRACK: *Create an ocean sound as you inhale and exhale, called* ujjayi *breathing, by slightly constricting the back of the throat, to help harness your attention to your breath.*

YOGA CONNECTION: *DIRGA PRANAYAMA* (THE THREE-PART BREATH)

Prana is the Sanskrit word for the "vital energy" or "life force" that animates all living beings. Yoga postures are designed to help facilitate a healthy flow of *prana* throughout the body, and yogic breathing practices, known as *pranayama*, are designed to enhance and regulate the flow of this vital energy. The basic yoga breathing practice of *Dirga Pranayama*, the Three-Part Breath, is particularly helpful for people in Western cultures, who tend to breathe shallowly only into the top part of the chest, because it teaches deep abdominal breathing, which completely fills the lungs on inhalation, providing the optimum amount of oxygen needed to nourish all cells of the body. In addition, when you bring air down into the lower portion of the lungs where oxygen exchange is most efficient, it triggers a cascade of relaxing physiologic changes: the heart rate slows, blood pressure decreases, muscles relax, anxiety eases, and the mind calms.

QUESTION

Is there any area of your body that feels closed or uncomfortable? Use your breath to release and cleanse any area of your body or spirit that needs attention.

Kavanah

Breath of life
Awaken my spirit
Fill my nostrils
Fill my lungs
Fill my soul
Give me a window
Into the pathways
That connect me to You
So that I may be open
To Your song

Personal Kavanah

_____

_____

_____

_____

2

אֱלֹהַי, נְשָׁמָה שֶׁנָתַתָּ בִּי טְהוֹרָה הִיא.

Elohai n'shamah shenatata bi t'horah hi.

The soul that you have given me, God, is pure.
Open up my heart to blessing.

Our offering of thanks to the Holy One for the purity of our soul, *Elohai N'shamah* appears in the very middle of *Birchot HaShachar*, the Morning Blessings. The prayer presents an image of our soul in God's hand, having been created, shaped, and had life breathed into it, for us and all living things, by the Holy One. This is a very personal prayer, guiding us to look deep within ourselves to seek purity and to listen to the still, small voice of the Eternal, as described by the prophet Isaiah, speaking to us and through us. We give thanks for God's protection of every living soul and for breath, which is our vehicle for life.

Each morning *when we rise from slumber we rejoice in the miracle of the daily restoration of our soul to our body. In expression of gratitude, we open our heart center to create acceptance in our spirit, releasing anger, judgments, competition, ego, and pride. Perhaps there is someone or something we feel closed off from or are uncomfortable confronting. As we open our heart, we feel the walls we have built up around us crumble away. Alternately, we take a few moments to gaze inward and become more connected with our inner life. We hear our inner voice telling us what our body and our soul need. This is embodied in the seated cat and cow poses. By synchronizing our movement with our breath, we help connect our mind and body, bringing energy into each cell and helping us release anything we don't need. Gazing inward, we connect to our innermost thoughts, focusing on what we do need. Inhaling and shining the light of the heart toward the sky, we lift and expand. Exhaling and softening the heart, we gaze inward, finding our inner truth. We continue our heart opening throughout our service, becoming ever more accepting of ourselves and aware of our blessings from God.*

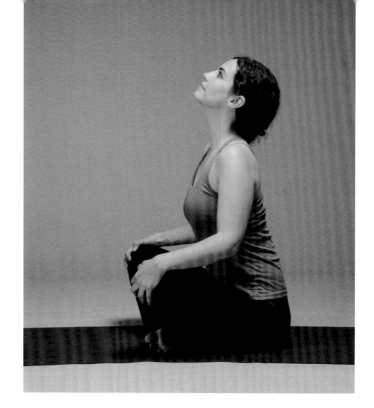

DIRECTIONS

Place your hands on your knees, and on an inhalation, draw your shoulder blades together, lifting the chest and shining the light of the heart upward, gazing toward the heavens, keeping length in the back of the neck (*top right*). While exhaling, hug your belly in

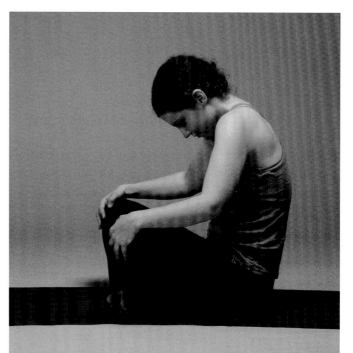

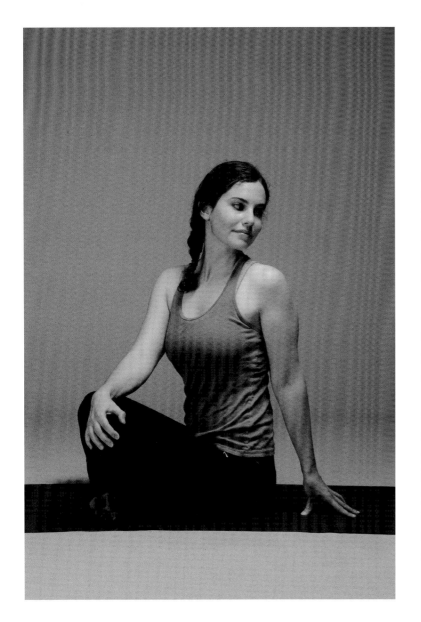

and release your chin to your chest, letting your shoulders relax, engaging you inner core, gazing inward (*facing page, bottom*). Once again on an inhalation, draw your shoulder blades together, opening and lifting the chest, and gaze upward, the eye of your heart to the sky. Exhaling, hug your belly in as you round your back, and drop your head forward, gazing inward. Continue with this movement, synchronized with the breath, as you inhale and exhale. Now bring your left hand down to the floor behind you, using this action to help create length in your spine (*left*). Inhale and lengthen, exhale and gently twist your body to the left. Inhale back to center. Exhale and bring your right hand behind you as you gently twist to the right. Continue this gentle twisting action, riding the waves of your breath.

ADVANCED TRACK: *Bring your arms back behind you with fingertips to the floor, opening your chest to the sky (appendix, fig. 2.1). Extend your arms forward, hinge from the hips, and bow your head toward the earth (appendix, fig. 2.2).*

CHAIR MODIFICATION: *Sitting tall with your hands on your thighs, inhale and lift your chest toward the sky. Gaze up but do not drop your head back; keep the back of your neck long (appendix, fig. 2.3). Exhale and return to sitting tall, releasing your chin to your chest and lifting your chest to your chin. If you have or are at risk for osteoporosis, avoid rounding your back as you drop your head forward—keep your spine long (appendix, fig. 2.4). Gently turn your body from side to side (appendix, fig. 2.5).*

YOGA CONNECTION: THE HEART CHAKRA

According to the yogic tradition, there are seven main energy centers, called "chakras," located along the spine. Literally translated as "wheel," a chakra is thought to be a kind of spinning vortex of energy that corresponds to a particular physical, mental, and energetic aspect of our being. The heart chakra, called *anahata*, is located in the center of the chest and is considered the seat of love and compassion. It is also thought to be a major hub of energy, in part due to its central location between the upper and lower body and between the right and left arm. This heart-opening sequence helps enhance the flow of energy and *prana* throughout the heart region.

QUESTION

What person, situation, or life challenge has caused you to shut down or close yourself off? Imagine the walls and defenses you've built up around your heart soften and melt away. Replace that feeling with acceptance.

KAVANAH

Open up my heart
And fill it full of blessing
Open up my spirit
So I may listen well
To the voice,
The still, small voice
Within.

Crumble away the fear
And forgive transgressions
Done in pain and anger
Redeemed through patience
Understanding
Awareness
And love.

PERSONAL KAVANAH

_____

_____

_____

3

נִשְׁמַת כָּל חַי תְּבָרֵךְ אֶת שְׁמִךָ.

Nishmat kol chai t'vareich et shimcha.

Let everything that has breath sing praises.
Sing songs of praise all the earth!

The next part of the morning service contains a series of psalm texts called *P'sukei D'zimrah*, which follow the Morning Blessings. The final of these praises (included only in the Shabbat and festival liturgy) is *Nishmat Kol Chai*, based on multiple psalm texts. It is an expression of exaltation and blessing of the Holy One, *Adonai*, the One who transcends time and space, God of all creatures and guide for life and power in the universe for all generations, past, present, and future. To this highest power *only* do we praise and exalt forever!

We conclude *our introductory prayers with praise and thanks for the multitude of miracles that bless our lives every day. We expand our connection with the life force of the planet as we become aware of sharing our prana, our life energy, with plants, animals, and other living things. We also become aware of the unseen energy and spiritual forces at work in the universe. From individual to community to the entire planet and even to the universe, our awareness of our interconnection with all beings continues to expand and evolve, encompassing a wider understanding of consciousness and spiritual awakening. Releasing our neck and upper body frees our energy flow, brings the circle of spirit into our physical being, and releases unwanted anger and anxiety from the throat.*

DIRECTIONS

Continue to root the sit bones down into the earth, with hands resting comfortably, heart lifted, and shoulders relaxed. Drop your right ear to your right shoulder (*right*). Release the muscles in the left side of the neck. Now gently drop your chin to your chest and roll your left ear to your left shoulder, releasing the muscles in the right side of the neck. Inhale while bringing your head back to center, then reverse the earlier action, dropping the left ear to the left shoulder, and continue this flow, keeping your breath slow and deep and even. Now bring your hands to your knees and begin to move your upper body in a large circle—forward, then to the right, to the back, then to the left—as if you were stirring a large pot. Continue to breathe as you enlarge this

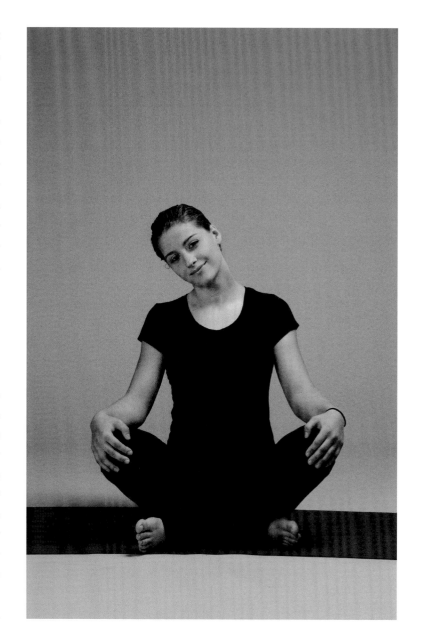

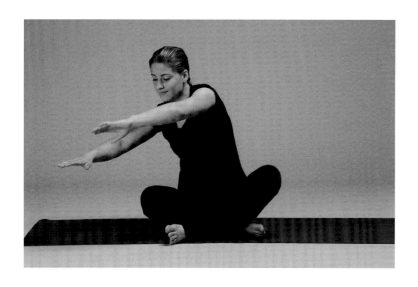

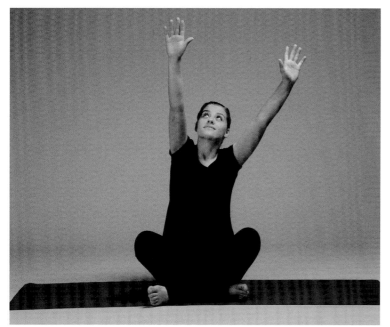

circle of spirit. Then, if it is possible for you to do so, sweep your arms up and around, making a large circle with your upper body and bringing your arms forward, brushing your fingertips to the floor (*top left*). When you're ready, stop your arms overhead and reverse direction (*bottom left*), sweeping your arms in a large circle as you bring an intention of praise for the circle of life into your body.

ADVANCED VARIATION: *Inhale and reach your arms up to the sky, palms forward, and gently hinge forward, bringing your hands or forearms to the ground in a sitting forward fold, releasing the muscles in the back and thighs (appendix, fig. 3.1). Coming up, switch the cross of your legs, and bring the opposite leg in front. Inhale, reach your arms up with palms forward, and hinge forward, bringing your hands or forearms to the floor in a sitting forward fold and releasing the muscles in the back and the opposite thigh. Continue to release and breathe as you let go of tension in your lower back and hips.*

CHAIR MODIFICATION: *If you have or are at risk for osteoporosis, do not round your back—circle your arms up and around as you breathe, keeping your spine extended (appendix, fig. 3.2).*

Question

Do you sense any unexpressed emotions in your throat? As you release your neck and shoulders, allow your throat to soften and relax.

YOGA CONNECTION: THE THROAT CHAKRA

In our high-stress, hurried, 24/7 world, neck and shoulder tension is common. Much of this pain is related to the postural stress of spending most of our days sitting, often doing activities that round our bodies forward—such as computer work, driving, and reading. Add to this the emotional tension of work deadlines, financial pressures, and caregiving responsibilities, and it's no wonder many people say the muscles in their upper back and neck are "hard as a rock." In addition, as the central channel connecting the head to the heart, the neck and shoulder region can be a bottleneck for emotional conflicts and spiritual struggles between what we think and what we feel. The throat chakra is the center of communication, associated with expressing yourself honestly and clearly speaking your truth. Conflicts between what we think and what we say—for example, if we lie or repress anger—are thought to lead to pain or disease in this area. If you've ever experienced a "lump" in your throat, you may appreciate this yogic view of how turbulent thoughts and emotions can express themselves physically. The neck and upper body flow are geared to relieving stiffness in this area, stretching muscles, and enhancing energy flow.

KAVANAH

When I praise
I ignite a spark in myself
Which allows me
To see the positive
To minimize the negative

To judge less
To accept more
To allow all the energy of the universe
To flow through me . . .
Rejoice!

PERSONAL KAVANAH

_____

_____

_____

_____

PART II
The *Sh'ma* and Its Blessings

CALL TO PRAYER: *Bar'chu* ✦ MUSIC: Craig Taubman

בָּרְכוּ אֶת יְיָ הַמְבֹרָךְ!
בָּרוּךְ יְיָ הַמְבֹרָךְ לְעוֹלָם וָעֶד!

Bar'chu et Adonai ham'vorach!
Baruch Adonai ham'vorach l'olam va-ed!

Praised be to Adonai! Holy Presence of the universe, we praise You now and forever!

The *Bar'chu* is known as the call to worship and is the first in a series of prayers called *Sh'ma Uvirchoteha*, the *Sh'ma* and Its Blessings, which prepares us for the recitation of the *Sh'ma*, the central prayer of the Jewish faith. We stand and face Jerusalem and the holy ark as we invoke praise to *Adonai*. It is traditional for the prayer leader to recite the call to prayer and for the congregation to respond. The prayer leader then repeats the call. The word *berech* in Hebrew means "knee," and Jews traditionally bow during the *Bar'chu* by bending the knees, then hinging forward from the hips on the word *Bar'chu*, and coming up on the word *Adonai*. In doing so, we acknowledge our service and humility before the Holy One.

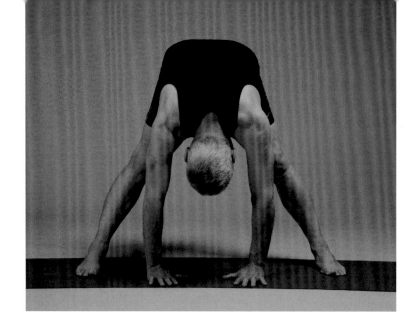

We've moved *from spiritual awareness of self to a broader spiritual awareness of all living things, and now during the* Bar'chu *we seek an understanding of a higher power in the universe. The act of bowing and prostration acknowledges this higher power and is an expression of our humility and readiness to accept that we cannot always be in control of our lives. This posture of release is a vulnerable one and helps us to prepare for the* Sh'ma. *Begin by tuning in to your breath and focusing on each inhalation and exhalation to bring you fully into the present moment. Imagine life-giving blood filling your veins and arteries, bringing oxygenated fluid to your brain, your upper body, and your organs. With each inhalation and exhalation in this inverted posture, let your shoulders, neck, and back release any unneeded burdens and stress. Picture tension, stress, and anything else you don't need falling away, replaced by calm and contentment.*

DIRECTIONS

Step your legs out wide and bring your hands to your lower back, fingers pointing toward the earth and elbows moving toward each other. Inhaling, lift your heart to the sky and gently arch your back. Exhaling, slide your hands down to the front of your thighs as you hinge forward from the hips with a long spine and bow forward (*top right*). Feel free to bend your knees if you like, or for more challenge, deepen your bow by releasing your hands down to your shins or ankles or to the floor. Invite your head to be

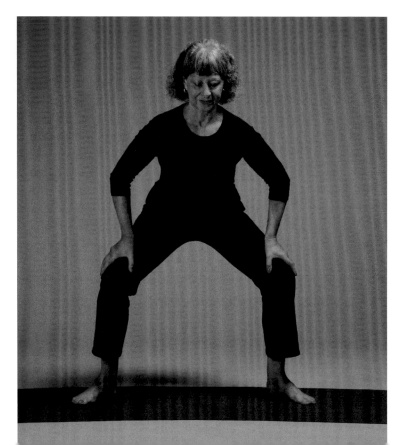

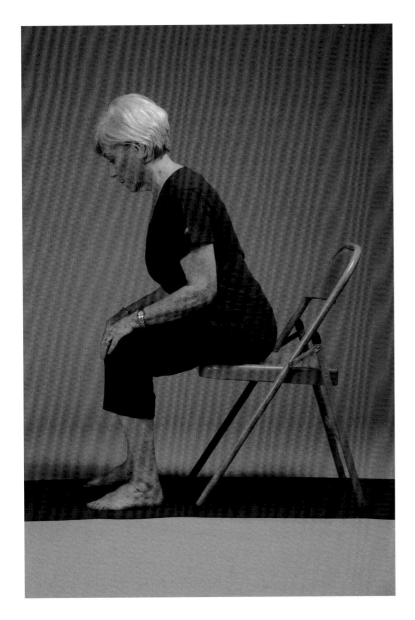

heavy so your neck and shoulders can relax and release. Breathe. As you are ready, inhale back up and step your feet into Mountain Pose, standing tall with feet hip-distance apart and hands down to your sides.

ADVANCED TRACK: *Bend forward and bring your elbows to the ground, keeping your knees straight and belly hugged in. Repeat this track again if you wish to give yourself additional time to experience the benefits of forward bend.*

GENTLE VARIATION: *If you have back pain and/or osteoporosis, keep your knees bent and your hands on your thighs as you hinge from the hips and bow forward with a flat back (facing page, bottom).*

CHAIR MODIFICATION: *From a seated position, bow forward from the hips, keeping your back straight and your spine long, and rest your forearms on your thighs (left).*

QUESTION

What is keeping you from being fully present today? Let your burdens fall away from your shoulders.

YOGA CONNECTION: FORWARD BENDS

Forward bending postures help calm the nervous system and are relaxing and introverted. The deep, standing forward bend, known as *Uttanasana* in Sanskrit, also carries the benefits of an inverted posture, since the head is below the heart. This position enhances blood flow to the brain and helps reverse the typical downward pull of gravity on the upper body.

KAVANAH

We bow in humility to You,
O High and Hidden One.
We acknowledge that we are not always in control
Even as we realize that while we are insignificant
Our lives uniquely matter.
Blessed are You, Holy Presence of the universe,
Our bodies sing Your praise!

PERSONAL KAVANAH

_____

_____

_____

_____

5

SUN SALUTATION: *Yotzeir Or* ✦ MUSIC: Folk Tune from Argentina

בָּרוּךְ אַתָּה יְיָ אֱלֹהֵינוּ מֶלֶךְ הָעוֹלָם יוֹצֵר
אוֹר וּבוֹרֵא חְשֶׁךְ עֹשֶׂה שָׁלוֹם וּבוֹרֵא
אֶת–הַכֹּל.

Baruch atah, Adonai, Eloheinu Melech haolam, yotzeir or uvorei choshech, oseh shalom uvorei et hakol.

Blessed are You, Holy Presence of the universe, Creator of light and darkness, Fashioner of all things.

Yotzeir Or is the second prayer in the series of prayers leading up to the *Sh'ma*. The first line is taken from Isaiah 45:7, praising the Holy One for forming light and creating darkness. The prayer goes on to praise God for making peace and fashioning all things as well as for wisdom in forming all the creatures of the earth. The theme of this prayer is light, illumination, and daily renewal as we continue the process of Creation. The final reflection of this prayer, making a return to Reform liturgy in *Mishkan T'filah*, highlights our devotion to the State of Israel: *Or chadash al Tzion ta-ir*, "Shine a new light upon Zion," our beacon of radiance and hope for the future.

The worship *of sun, moon, and stars was integral to many ancient cultures. In Judaism, we instead praise God as the creator of the heavenly bodies. God's role in Creation is a focal point for preparing to recite the* Sh'ma, *the holiest of holy prayers we know. From the vulnerability and humility of the* Bar'chu, *we move to an awareness of our place in the larger universe and our partnership with God in the repair of our world,* tikkun olam. *The Sun Salutation Flow is our call to action. It challenges us physically while focusing our intention on what it is we are called to do. As we move through this* Vinyasa, *or linked series of yoga postures, we link ourselves to the process of Creation.*

DIRECTIONS

There are two options for this sequence. For Sun Salutation Flow, begin in Mountain Pose (*right*), then inhale as you bring your arms up, palms facing each other, gazing up (*facing page, left*). Then exhale and sweep them out and down as you swan-dive forward, bringing the fingertips to the floor in a forward fold (*facing page, top right*). Inhale and step your right foot (*facing page, bottom right*) and then your left foot back, then exhale as you lift your hips and press back into Downward-Facing Dog Pose (*page 32, left*). Inhale and shift your weight forward into Plank Pose (*page 32, right*). Exhale and lower yourself down onto your belly (*page 33, left*); then inhale and open your heart into Cobra Pose, keeping your elbows tucked in close to your body and your neck extended, gazing forward (*page 33, right*). Exhale as you

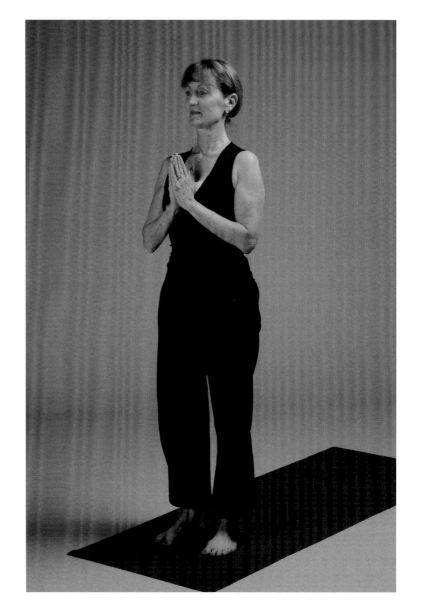

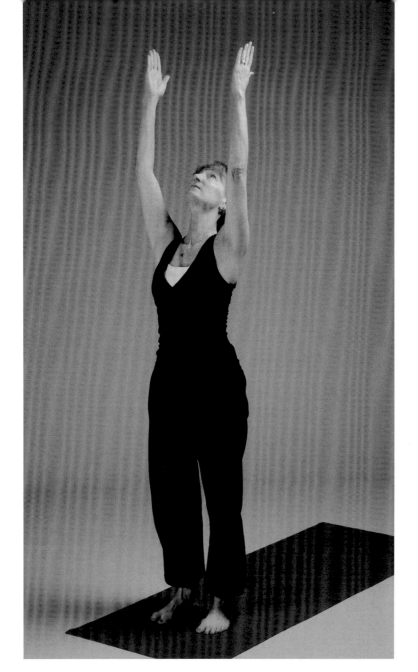

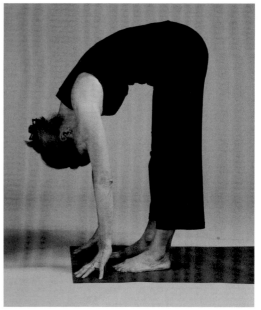

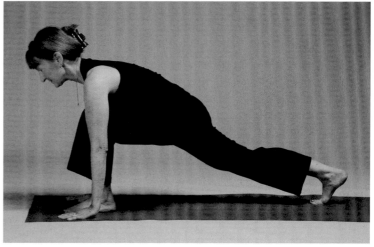

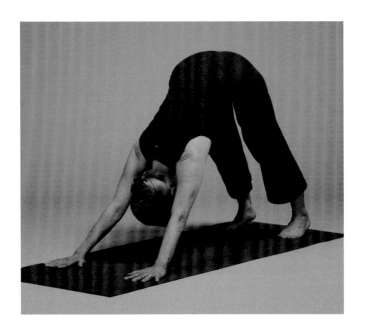

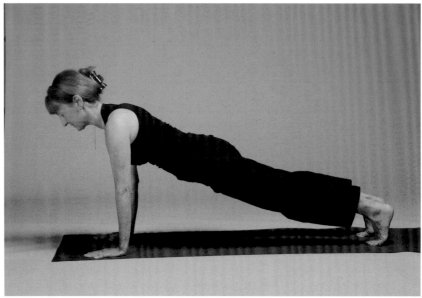

push the floor away and press back into Downward-Facing Dog Pose. Inhale and lift your right leg up, flexing your foot, look toward your hands, and bring your right foot between your hands (*appendix, fig. 5.1*). Exhale and step your left foot to meet the right. Inhale as you lift back up into Mountain Pose while bringing your arms up and away from your body with your palms together overhead. Exhale and move your hands down to heart center (*appendix, fig. 5.2*). Do that flow twice more.

For a simpler flow, come to standing, feet hip-width apart in Mountain Pose, then inhale as you step forward with your right foot, front knee bent and arms extended up (*appendix, fig. 5.3*). This is Warrior I Pose. Exhale as you step the right foot back to

Mountain Pose. Inhale and step the left foot forward, front knee bent and arms extended up, to Warrior Pose. Exhale as you step the left foot back to Mountain Pose. Inhale as you step out to the right, toes pointed outward, right knee bent and arms extended out at shoulder height (*appendix, fig. 5.4*). This is Warrior II Pose. Exhale as you step your right foot back to Mountain Pose. Inhale as you step your left foot out to the left, toes pointed outward, left knee bent and arms extended out at shoulder height. Exhale as you step back to Mountain Pose. Inhale as you step back on your right foot and bring your arms up overhead, again coming into Warrior I Pose and gently bending backward with the front knee bent. Exhale as you bring the right foot back to Mountain Pose. Inhale as you step back with your left foot, front knee bent

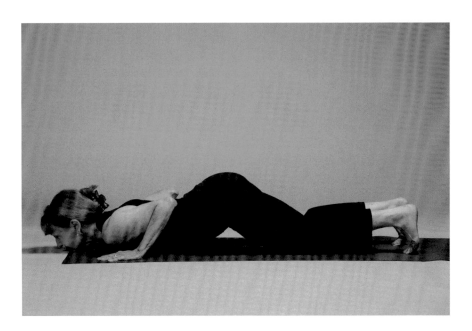

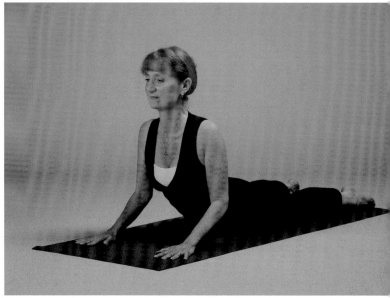

and arms extended up overhead, gently bending backward. Step your left foot back to Mountain Pose. Extend your arms out in a wide sweep to the sides, all the way up overhead and then in a wide sweep down to your sides. Repeat this sequence two more times.

CHAIR MODIFICATION: *Sit tall in your chair and as you inhale, bring your arms out and up, palms together, gazing up (appendix, fig. 5.5). As you exhale, bring your hands straight down the center line of the body, resting at the heart (appendix, fig. 5.6). As an additional variation, you can add the arm portion of the Warrior Flow (appendix, fig. 5.7).*

YOGA CONNECTION: SURYA NAMASKAR

The Sun Salutation Flow, or *Surya Namaskar*, is a classic sequence of yoga postures thought to originate in ancient practices of sun worship. While the specific postures used in the sequence may vary slightly, depending on the style or school of yoga, virtually all versions of the Sun Salutation Flow can be used as a practice in itself—stretching and strengthening the body's major muscle groups, flexing and extending the spine, and creating an aerobic effect with continuous repetition.

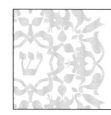

QUESTION

What role do you play in repairing the world? Envision yourself as God's partner.

KAVANAH

When I falter, give me strength
When others are in need
Bring my hands to help
Adonai
Guide my body in strength
Help me to light the way for good.

PERSONAL KAVANAH

_____

_____

_____

_____

_____

_____

6

בָּרוּךְ אַתָּה יְיָ הַבּוֹחֵר בְּעַמּוֹ יִשְׂרָאֵל
בְּאַהֲבָה.

Baruch atah, Adonai, habocheir b'amo Yisrael b'ahavah.

Blessed are You, Adonai, who has chosen our people Israel in love.

Ahavah Rabbah, another in the series of prayers that prepare us for the recitation of the *Sh'ma,* means "great love" and introduces the theme of God's love for the Jewish people, which is continued through the next few prayers of our service. It challenges us to follow in the footsteps of our ancestors, trusting the Holy One to teach us the lessons and rules that are important and helping us to understand deeper meaning of those rules in our lives. The Torah, the master guide for these laws, is mentioned twice in the prayer, focusing our attention on the mitzvot, or commandments, that will lead us to a life of joy and peace.

In final preparation *for the* Sh'ma, *our prayer of prayers, we create a* kavanah, *or intention, for ourselves today. Consider why you are here. What has brought you to your mat, your* mishkan, *your holy place? Are you seeking peace of mind, or strength of body? Perhaps you are seeking an escape from the burdens of everyday life and are looking for more balance or contentment of spirit. Your* kavanah *serves as a focal point for your energy, helping to harness your mind for positive change. We create this* kavanah *as a gift to ourselves that we will use throughout our worship practice and allow to carry over into our daily lives. Just as we say a blessing before the study of Torah, we spend a moment to reflect on our* kavanah *for the day.*

DIRECTIONS

From Mountain Pose, with feet hip-distance apart, root down through the soles of the feet and take a full, deep breath as you extend the top of your head toward the heavens. Engage the muscles in the front of your thighs so they hug the bone, draw your belly in toward your spine, and relax your shoulders down away from your ears. Bring your hands to your heart center. On an inhalation, bend your knees and hinge slightly forward from your hips—keeping your spine long—as you drop your bottom down as if you were about to sit in an imaginary chair (*right*); this is known as Chair Pose). Bring your arms forward and up, palms facing inward, as though you were holding an imaginary ball. Let that ball contain your blessing for yourself today. Then, exhale as

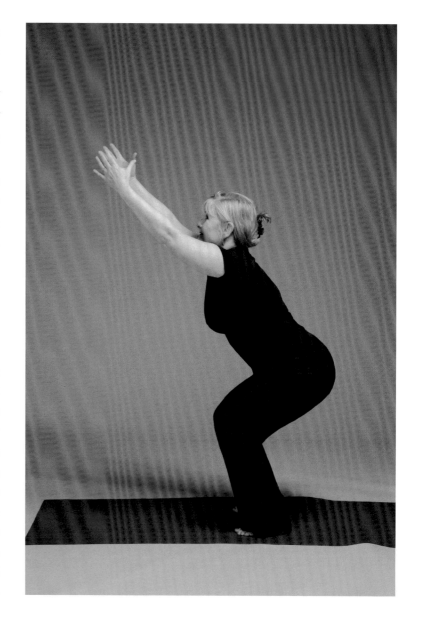

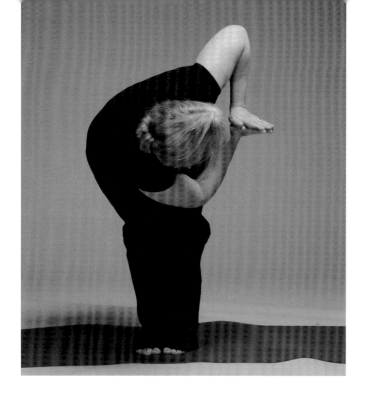

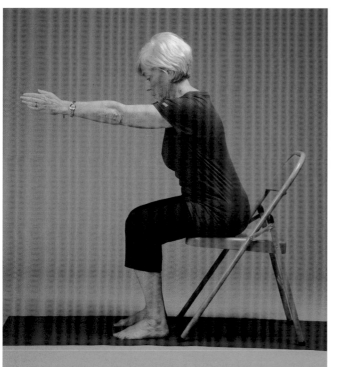

you stand back up into Mountain Pose, relaxing your arms down, then inhale back to Chair Pose. Flow back and forth between these two postures, moving with your breath. If you'd like extra challenge, stay in Chair Pose through a complete breath cycle or more, sinking deeper into the pose with each breath.

ADVANCED VARIATION: *From Chair Pose, bring your hands to prayer, then fold forward and bring your left elbow to the outside of the right knee, using this action to twist right and look up to the sky* (top left). *Stay here for several breaths, and then switch sides.*

GENTLE VARIATION: *In Chair Pose, lift your arms to shoulder height.*

CHAIR MODIFICATION: *Hinge forward from the hips, keeping the spine long and extend the arms forward* (bottom left).

QUESTION

What is your intention for your practice today? Fill your mind with what you wish to accomplish.

YOGA CONNECTION: *SAMKALPA*

An important part of the yoga practice is clarifying your intention, a process known as *samkalpa*. Like a New Year's resolution, a *samkalpa* is a desire or wish that you clearly state or affirm to help channel your energies to move in a particular direction. This concept recognizes the importance of the mind-body connection and highlights yoga's power to harness the mind for healing and spiritual development. If you aimlessly step onto your yoga mat and mindlessly move through the motions, the result is likely to be quite different, and less effective, than if you set an intention for your practice and then move diligently along your chosen path.

KAVANAH

We prepare our minds for the *Sh'ma*
With purpose and intention
Strong in our desire
To embody truth
Molding ourselves into
The reality that we wish to create
Reaching toward the sky for
The possibilities of what our spirit knows

Whispers of hope
But only beginning to understand
The message bubbling forth
A prayer only for ourselves
An epiphany
Like the wisdom written in its verses
Torah speaking through us
Will we listen?

PERSONAL KAVANAH

_____

_____

_____

7

TOWARD ONENESS: *Sh'ma* ✦ MUSIC: "Listen" by Ira Fein

שְׁמַע יִשְׂרָאֵל יְהוָה אֱלֹהֵינוּ יְהוָה אֶחָד!

Sh'ma Yisrael, Adonai Eloheinu, Adonai Echad!

Listen, listen . . . to One within. Listen to the One . . . deep within your soul.

Taken from a verse in the Torah, Deuteronomy 6:4, we recite the *Sh'ma* to bear witness to the Oneness of God. The *Sh'ma* is often referred to as "the watchword of our faith," and the central idea of the belief in One God has distinguished Judaism from other religions. It is an imperative for Israel to listen and hear it declared that *Adonai* alone is our God. The theme of love surrounds this prayer, both in the *Ahavah Rabbah*, recited before the *Sh'ma*, and the *V'ahavta*, which is chanted immediately following it. It is customary in Reform congregations to stand during the recitation of the *Sh'ma*, but in other synagogues the prayer is recited sitting. Traditionally, it is recited three times a day, often with eyes covered or closed in order to heighten concentration on the powerful words and block outside distractions.

With our kavanah *in our thoughts and pure intention in our heart, we blend the awareness of Divine Presence in the expansive universe into a single intention of Oneness: mind, body, and spirit. We listen to the beat of our hearts, allowing this miraculous pumping to fill us with quietness, wholeness, and peace. To embody Oneness, we imagine our arms form the Hebrew letter* yod, *two yods representing the name of God. Extending our limbs out from our body, we mold ourselves into the letter* alef, *which begins each Hebrew word:* Adonai* Eloheinu, Adonai Echad, "Adonai *is our God,* Adonai *is One."*

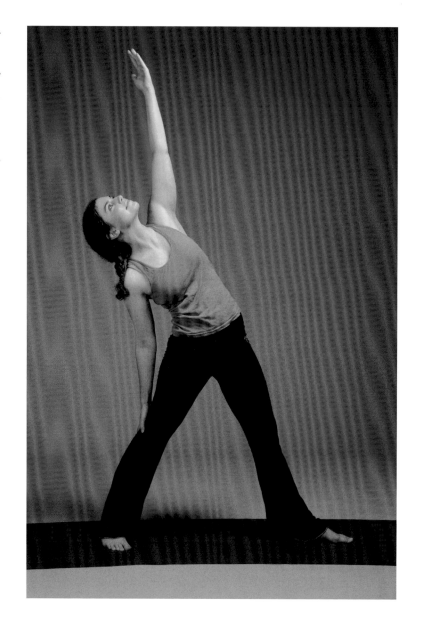

DIRECTIONS

Come into a comfortably wide stance, and turn your right foot out to ninety degrees as you turn your left foot in to a forty-five-degree angle. On an inhalation, extend your arms out to the sides, palms down. On an exhalation, relax your shoulders down away from your ears. Inhaling, turn your head to gaze over the middle finger of your right hand. Exhaling, hinge from the hips as you gently bend over your front leg, allowing your right hand to rest wherever it is comfortable on your right leg as your left arm extends up toward the sky (*right*); this is known as Triangle Pose. Keep the breath flowing, and if you like, turn your gaze up toward your left hand. Inhale as you move back up to a standing

---

* The Hebrew is actually יהוה, the tetragrammaton, which stands in for the name of God and which we pronounce as "Adonai," אֲדֹנָי.

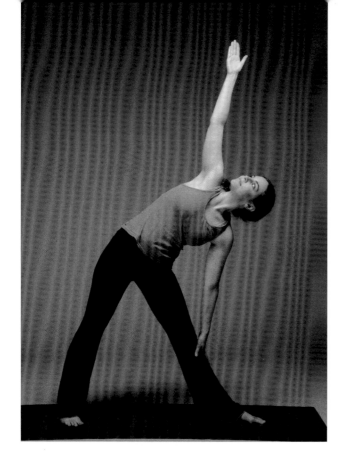

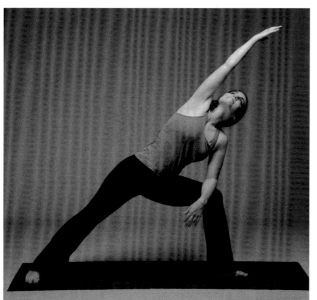

position, then exhale as you bring your left hand to your left thigh and your right hand up toward the sky (*top left*). Do this several times, hinging back and forth between Triangle and Reverse Triangle. Then switch sides and repeat this flow. Walk your legs back together and bring your hands to heart center.

ADVANCED TRACK: *From Triangle Pose, bend the front knee, extend the body forward, place the front forearm on the front thigh, and sweep the back arm up and over into Side Angle Pose (bottom left).*

GENTLE VARIATION: *Step your feet out wide, with toes angled out. Place your left hand on your hip and extend your right arm up overhead as you sidebend to the left. Stay here for a few breaths, then switch sides (appendix, fig. 7.1). Place your left hand on the left thigh and extend the right arm up, and gaze at your palm as you gently arch back (appendix, fig. 7.2). Stay here for a few breaths, then switch sides.*

CHAIR MODIFICATION: *Place your left hand on your left hip, extend your right arm up, and gently sidebend to the left (appendix, fig. 7.3). Stay here for a few breaths, then switch sides.*

QUESTION

When you listen to the One, what do you hear? Is there a voice within that speaks to you?

YOGA CONNECTION: MANTRA

A mantra is a thought or intention expressed as a sound or phrase that is used as a focus of meditation. Typically, a mantra is repeated over and over again, silently or aloud. Repetition of a mantra helps focus the mind, so the practitioner becomes absorbed in the sound. One well-known mantra is the syllable "om," considered by Hindus to be a sacred syllable representing the ultimate reality. This syllable is part of the word *shalom*, which is often used as a mantra by Jewish yoga practitioners.

KAVANAH

When our people
Was called
To listen
We heard the voice
Of the Eternal
Speaking in our hearts
To believe
In what we could not see
To hope
In what we could not touch
And thus

We found the courage
To know that You exist.
In us,
In others,
In nature,
In spirit.
Seen and unseen
Tangible and intangible
Unifying
Oneness.

PERSONAL KAVANAH

_____

_____

_____

8

STRENGTH AND FREEDOM: *Mi Chamochah* ✦ MUSIC: Bonia Shur

מִי־כָמְכָה בָּאֵלִם יְיָ? מִי כָּמְכָה נֶאְדָּר בַּקֹּדֶשׁ?
נוֹרָא תְהִלֹּת, עֹשֵׂה פֶלֶא.
יְיָ יִמְלֹךְ לְעוֹלָם וָעֶד.

Mi chamochah ba-elim Adonai? Mi kamochah nedar bakodesh?
Nora t'hilot, oseh feleh. Adonai yimloch l'olam va-ed.

Who is like You, O Eternal One, among all the powers of the universe?
Holy One of Blessing, strengthen and free us.

Mi Chamochah comes from Exodus 15:11, within the poetic verses of *Shirat HaYam*, the Song at the Sea. When the Isra-elites fleeing Egypt successfully crossed the Sea of Reeds, Miriam, Moses's sister, took up her timbrel and led our people in this song of rejoicing, which has remained in our liturgy to remind us daily of our enslavement in Egypt and our ultimate flight to free-dom. Its themes of praise, gratitude, and redemption remind us of God's promise to support and strengthen us in times of need.

Warrior Poses embody *our transition from slavery to freedom. Long ago our people were enslaved in Egypt, forced to live a life of hard labor and degradation. Today the fast pace of modern life has enslaved us in many other ways—to our careers, our activities, our computers, our smart phones, and various other addictions. We may even be enslaved by our own inability to break free of whatever is hurting us. Warrior I Pose helps us find the strength to change the things in our lives that are in our power to change. Feel the power of the Warrior fill your being as you sense your ability to cope with the challenges of everyday life and free yourself from what is holding you captive. Warrior II Pose opens our heart and helps us attain the flexibility to accept the things in our life we cannot change. Our heart expands and softens, and our mind remains open to new possibilities for accepting the things that are inevitable. We are free from self-doubt and indecision. Reverse Warrior helps us to reflect on what battles we wish to fight and which are best relinquished.*

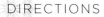

DIRECTIONS

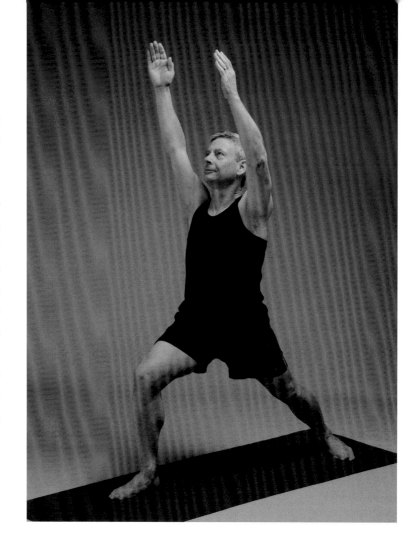

Stand at the back of your mat, and step your right foot forward, allowing the toes of your back foot to turn out slightly to the left. Imagine that each foot is on a train track (not a tightrope) so that your stance is wide and stable. Inhale and lengthen your body up through the crown of your head; then exhale and bend your right knee, being sure that it tracks directly forward over your toes. Inhaling, extend your arms up toward the sky, palms facing in.

Exhale and release your shoulders down away from your ears, forming Warrior I Pose (*above*). Stay here for several breaths, then open your arms and open your hips, bringing your right arm forward and left arm back to form Warrior II Pose (*facing page, left*). Be sure to keep the front knee pointing in the same direction as the front toes. Gaze over the fingertips of your front hand. Now turn your right palm up as you raise your right arm up over-

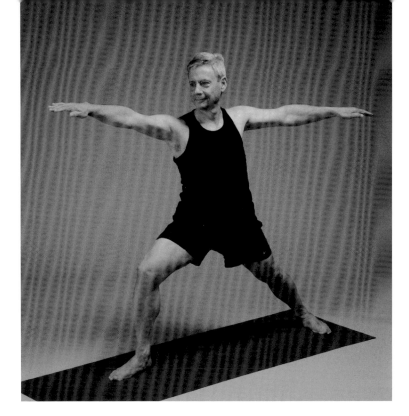

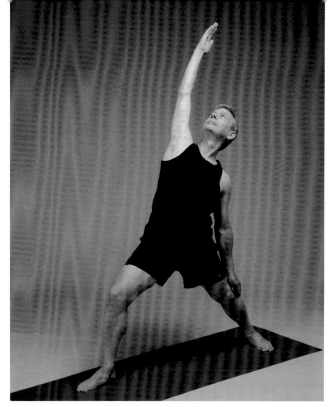

head and arch your back. Gazing up, let your left hand rest on your left thigh, moving into Reverse Warrior (*above, right*). Come back to Warrior II and step your right foot back and release. Move to the back of your mat and repeat this Warrior flow on the other side, stepping out with your left foot. When you reach the section of the prayer that begins *Tzur Yisrael*, come into Mountain Pose and lift your arms straight up to the sky, palms facing inward in Volcano Pose (*appendix, fig. 8.1*). Breathe as you visualize a white light entering your fingertips and feel a bolt of renewing energy flow down through your arms, elbows, upper arms, heart center, belly, abdomen, legs, knees, ankles, and feet. Bring your hands to Prayer Pose in front of your chest as you bring that energy into your heart center.

ADVANCED TRACK: *From Warrior I, propel yourself off the ball of the back foot and hinge forward, lifting the back leg off the ground and reaching forward into Warrior III. When you're ready, bring the back leg down. Go back into Warrior I to push off the ball of the opposite foot, reaching forward and lifting the back leg off the ground.*

GENTLE VARIATION: *Step your legs into Warrior I, and allow your elbows to bend into "cactus arms" (appendix, fig. 8.2).*

CHAIR MODIFICATION: *Step one foot forward and extend the arms into the Warrior positions (appendix, fig. 8.3).*

YOGA CONNECTION: WARRIOR POSES

Named for the mythical warrior Virabhadra, three basic standing postures (typically called Warrior I, II, and III or *Virabhadrasana* I, II, and III) help cultivate a sense of power, courage, and inner strength. Physically, the postures help strengthen the legs, back, shoulders, and arms while toning the abdominal muscles and opening the hips, groin, and chest. Energetically, these poses help build stamina and confidence. Modern yogis often consider themselves spiritual warriors, fighting the foe of *avidya*, or ignorance of the true nature of reality, which is a root cause of suffering.

QUESTION

What in your life enslaves you? What must you accept? Visualize change and acceptance in your life.

KAVANAH

It takes courage
To face life's challenges
It takes understanding
To accept life's unfairness
Just as the Israelites
Left Egypt with faith as their weapon
So do we
Harness our inner strength
To navigate tumultuous

Moments in our lives
Adapting, changing, coping, growing
Challenging ourselves
To rise, to overcome our demons,
To accept our inevitabilities
And to rejoice,
Each and every day
In our endeavors.

PERSONAL KAVANAH

_____

_____

_____

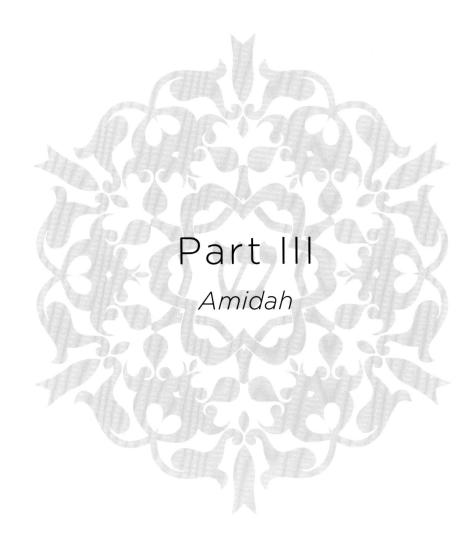

Part III

Amidah

אֲדוֹנָי, שְׂפָתַי תִּפְתָּח, וּפִי יַגִּיד תְּהִלָּתֶךָ.

Adonai, s'fatai tiftach, ufi yagid t'hilatecha.

Adonai, open my lips that I may find my way to You. Hallelujah!

The *Amidah* is the central portion of our worship service and is among the oldest prayer rubrics we know. The *Amidah* includes three themes: praises, petitions, and prayers for peace. The first section begins with the *Avot v'Imahot* prayer, which praises God for God's love of past, present, and future generations. The next prayer, *G'vurot*, describes the power of *Adonai* and references the divine ability to reverse death, a concept that has been transformed by Reform Judaism to extol God as the giver of life. The final prayer in this opening section of the *Amidah* is called *K'dushah*, meaning "holiness," during which we raise ourselves up on our toes when reciting *Kadosh, kadosh, kadosh*, "Holy, holy, holy" (Isaiah 6:3), bringing ourselves closer to heaven and the Divine Presence. The repetition *Adonai S'fatai* at the beginning of the *Amidah* is taken from Psalm 51:17, praising the Holy One for opening our lips to utter prayer.

Our worship journey *now calls us closer to the Ineffable, invitingus to speak directly with God through the embodiment of praise, power, and holiness. We remember that we are a link in a long chain of ancestors and traditions that date back thousands of years. By recalling their spirits, we connect with their energy, understand their journey, and visualize ourselves as an extension of their experiences. Our connection deepens as we stretch our bodies, feet firmly planted on the ground, allowing memories to move through us, in us, strengthening and supporting us. We channel that energy as we fill our bodies with the power we have been granted through the efforts and actions of others. We are filled with a sense of thanksgiving, strength, and well-being as we move ourselves closer to heaven and to the spirits that speak in us and through us every day. Bring to mind someone who is no longer with you upon whose shoulders you stand, and sense his or her spirit swirling in and around you as you move through these standing postures of praise.*

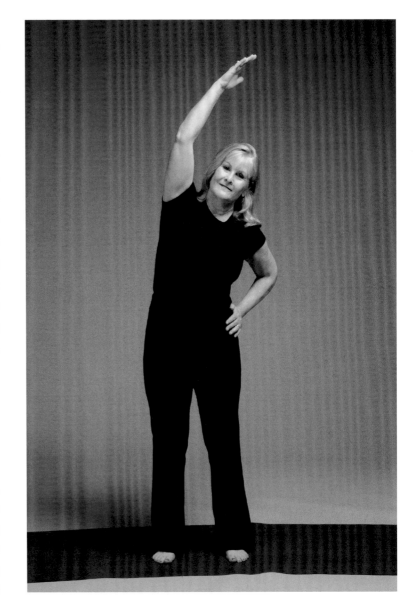

DIRECTIONS

Standing tall in Mountain Pose, bring your hands to your hips. Inhaling, extend your right arm out and up. Exhale as you gently side-bend over to the left, keeping both sides of your waist long (*right*). Stay here for a few breaths, then inhale back to Mountain Pose and repeat to the other side. If you like, continue flowing back and forth a few times. Now inhale and bring both arms up

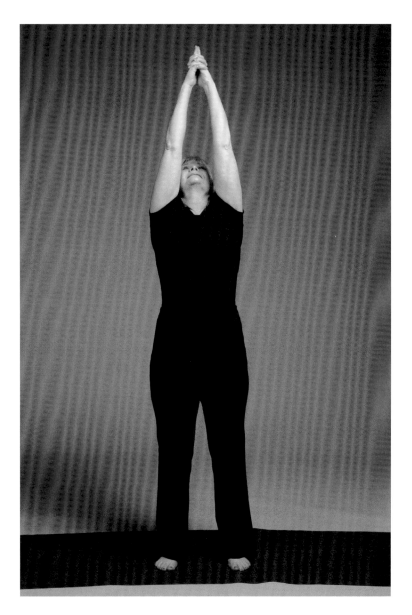

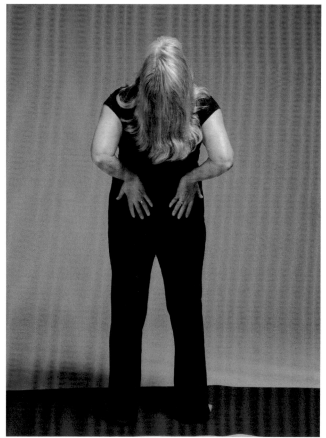

over your head, index fingers together with your other fingers intertwined (*top left*). As you stretch heavenward, lift your heels off the ground on an inhalation, then exhale and come down. Repeat two more times. Now release your arms out and bring them behind you, clasping your hands together and opening your heart to the sky (*top right*). Take a full breath and release your arms into

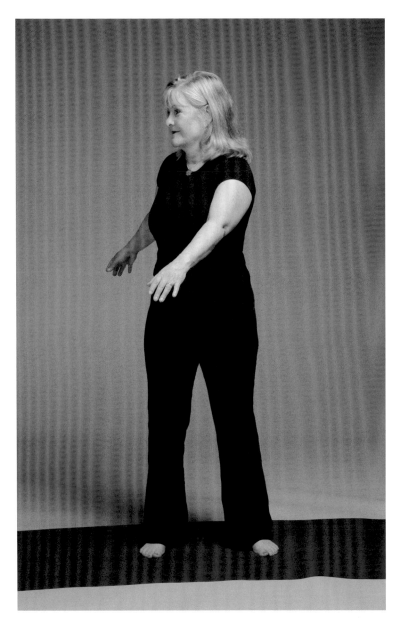

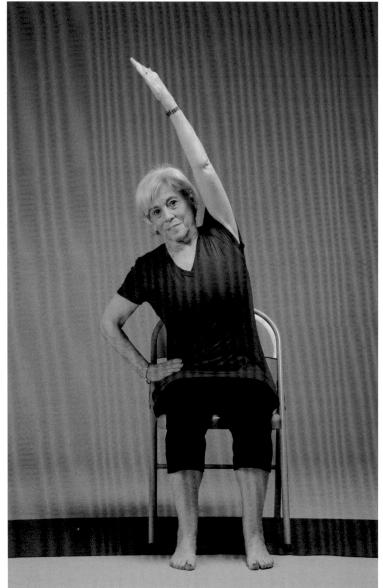

a "Y" shape, or Hallelujah Arms. Swing your hips and arms from side to side for a few breaths; then slowly bring your arms down, continuing to sway from side to side as you return to Mountain Pose (*facing page, left*).

CHAIR MODIFICATION: *Place your right hand on your right hip and extend your left arm out to the side, then up overhead. Inhale as you lengthen the spine. Exhale as you sidebend gently to the right (*facing page, right*). Switch sides.*

YOGA CONNECTION: THE SIDE BODY

Many activities of daily life bend the spine forward—working at a desk, driving, cooking, picking up a package or a child. Few routine actions involve side bending, which is why including lateral bends in a yoga practice is an important way to help strengthen the muscles in the torso, enhancing the flexibility of the side body. Be sure to avoid the common mistake of "crunching" over to one side; instead, focus on keeping both sides of the body lengthened during side-bending postures.

QUESTION

Who is the person no longer with you who has most influenced your life? Why? Picture his/her spirit moving through you.

Kavanah

There are people
We meet in our dreams
Deep pools of memory
A voice, a gesture, a movement
The color of an eye
Sparkling true
An accent
Speaking in a way that is familiar
We see hands grasping ours
Drawing us to the past
There, just beyond our worldly vision
A spirit standing next to us
We speak

Thinking we'll hear an answer
To a question we've always asked
What's for dinner?
Can I have that recipe?
Ones no longer with us
In our heads all the time!
Encouraging us to become
All we want to be
Speaking through us
And whispering the answers
To all our hidden questions
Sometimes knowing us better
Than we know ourselves.

Personal Kavanah

_____

_____

_____

_____

_____

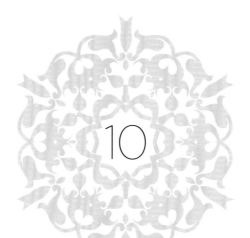

10

בָּרוּךְ אַתָּה יְיָ שׁוֹמֵעַ תְּפִלָּה.

Baruch atah Adonai shomei-a t'filah.

How blessed is this place: Adonai, Shechinah, *hear my prayer.*

The middle part of the *Amidah* consists of thirteen petitions for blessings on many different themes, including gaining wisdom, forgiveness, healing, abundance, freedom, justice, piety, and Jerusalem. The series of petitions ends with *Sh'ma koleinu:* "Hear our prayer, *Adonai.* Blessed are You who hears our prayer." On Shabbat all of these petitions are condensed into one prayer, *K'dushat HaYom,* which contains the *Yism'chu, V'shamru,* and *R'tzeih vim'nuchateinu,* prayers in celebration of the joy and sacredness of Shabbat. They are followed by two final prayers, *R'tzeih (Avodah)* and *Modim (Hodaah),* asking for acceptance of our prayers and giving thanks for the many miracles in our lives that we experience every day. Reform Jews generally recite these prayers seated.

This portion of the Amidah *is embodied on our mats, with our hands and knees connected to the earth. As we prostrate our bodies, we are again humbled and reminded of the many miracles and blessings in our lives that afford us relative comfort and ease. And yet this is the time in our service when we ask God for what we need in our lives, what we may be missing. These core strengthening postures help connect us to our center—to that deep, inner place of understanding and wisdom, which leads us to the truth that our body knows and our mind has yet to realize. Inner peace comes when we reveal the truths deep inside. We allow that knowledge to flow through us as we move through these intense and engaging floor poses. We also take a few moments to use these postures of blessing to petition for healing for our planet, the Land of Israel, or someone who is in need of our prayers.*

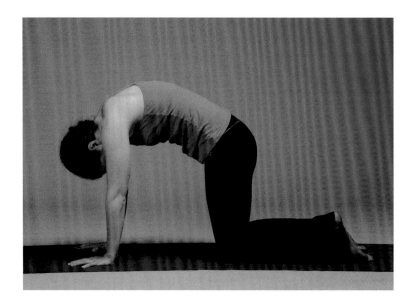

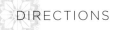

DIRECTIONS

Come onto your hands and knees, placing your wrists directly under your shoulders and your knees directly under your hips. Take a moment to make sure your weight is evenly divided among all four limbs. As you're ready, take a deep breath in and feel your rib cage expand all the way around. On an exhalation, arch your body up, dropping the head and dropping the tailbone. This is Cat Pose (*right*). On an inhalation, reverse the curve, so your spine drops down and your gaze lifts up, moving through the heart center. This is Cow Pose (*facing page, left*). Continue a few times, mov-

ing with the breath—exhaling to Cat, then inhaling to Cow. Then, from hands and knees position with your back flat—called Table Pose (*facing page, right*)—inhale the right arm forward and the left leg back, into Spinal Balance Pose (*appendix, fig. 10.1*), then exhale back to Table. Inhale the left arm forward and the right leg back into Spinal Balance, then exhale back to Table. Continue a few times at your own pace, holding the balance through a breath cycle if you like. Now begin to circle your hips to the right, creating a figure eight with your entire body. Stop and return to Table Pose, then circle to the left, continuing to flow and releasing your spine and hips. Next, from Table Pose, tuck your toes under and lift your hips to the sky, pressing your "paws" into the ground as you extend your "tail" back into Downward-Facing Dog Pose. Then shift your weight forward and drop your hips into a push-up position—this is called Plank Pose. Next, bend your elbows

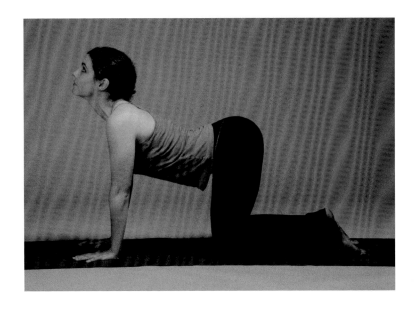

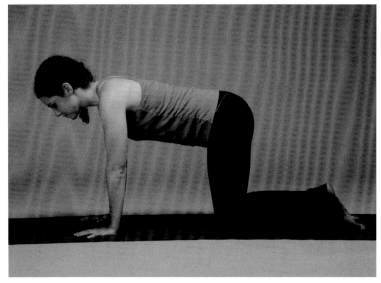

and slowly lower yourself onto your belly. Stack your palms and rest your forehead or your chin on the back of your hands. This is Crocodile Pose (*appendix, fig. 10.2*). Enjoy three full breaths here. Now root down through your pubic bone, and on an inhalation, lift your right leg up and reach it back. This is Modified Locust Pose (*appendix, fig. 10.3*). Exhale it back down, then inhale your left leg up and back, then exhale it back down. Continue a few more times, moving with your breath, then rest. Next, bring your elbows under your shoulders and extend your forearms forward, parallel to each other, palms down. Press your pubic bone down as you lift your chest, gazing forward and opening your heart center. This is Sphinx Pose (*appendix, fig. 10.4*). Stay here for a few breaths, allowing your heart to lift with each inhalation, rooting down with your legs on each exhalation. Focus your mind on whatever you are asking for today.

ADVANCED TRACK: *Lying on your belly, bend your knees, reach back with your arms, and hold your ankles or feet. On an inhalation, move your feet away from your buttocks and allow that action to lift your upper body up. Stay here for several slow, deep breaths, then relax and release.*

CHAIR MODIFICATION: *Sit tall in your chair with your palms on your thighs. On an inhalation, press down with your palms as you lift your heart up toward the sky in a seated backbend (appendix, fig. 10.5). On an exhalation, return to sitting tall, releasing your chin to your chest and lifting your chest to your chin (appendix, fig. 10.6). Avoid rounding your back. Continue several times. Next, inhale while lifting your right arm and extending your left leg forward (appendix, fig. 10.7), then exhale while moving back to the starting position. Repeat on the other side.*

YOGA CONNECTION: ANIMAL POSTURES

Yoga poses are frequently named for animals, such as Cat, Cow, Crocodile, and Locust in this sequence. It is thought that the sages who developed the posture practice looked to nature for inspiration and modeled some movements on those observed in the animal kingdom. Other common postures with animal names include Cobra, Frog, Heron, Rabbit, Fish, Eagle, Lion, and Crow.

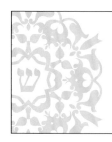

QUESTION

What does the world need today? Use these postures to feel empowered to ask for what is needed in the world.

KAVANAH

How can I ask
For clarity and truth
For what is needed in the world
When so much in the world
Is broken?
How can I reconcile
Needing
When so many are in need?
I feel powerless
To fix, to heal and repair

And yet
My prayers
Help heal
What is broken
In me
So that I may do
For others
And in a way
That is everything.

PERSONAL KAVANAH

_____

_____

_____

11

MEDITATIONS OF THE HEART: *Elohai N'tzor* ✦ MUSIC: "Y'hi-yu l'ratzon" by Danny Maseng

יִהְיוּ לְרָצוֹן אִמְרֵי פִי וְהֶגְיוֹן לִבִּי לְפָנֶיךָ,
יְיָ צוּרִי וְגוֹאֲלִי.

Yih'yu l'ratzon imrei fi v'hegyon libi l'fanecha, Adonai tzuri v'go-ali.

*May the prayers of my mouth and intentions of my heart
be true to all that is within me.*

The final section of the *Amidah* consists of three prayers for peace and concludes this section of our service. The first, *Sim Shalom*, is a petition: "Grant peace, goodness and blessing, grace, kindness, and mercy, to us and all Your people Israel" (Elyse D. Frishman, ed., *Mishkan T'filah* [New York: CCAR, 2007]). The second, *Elohai N'tzor*, based on Psalms 34:14, 60:7, and 19:15, asks *Adonai* in a very personal way "to guard my speech from evil and my lips from deception" (*Mishkan T'filah*). The transition from communal petition to asking for oneself is marked by silence and time for thoughts and meditations. The *Amidah* is completed by the singing of *Oseh Shalom*, "May the One who makes peace in the high heavens, send peace to us and all the world."

The central part *of our service ends with a personal prayer of the heart. We are not praising, nor are we asking for anything. We are simply letting the intentions of our prayers settle in our heart center, resonating and filling us with inner peace and rest. In Child's Pose, we relinquish and restore, relax and release any distracting and disquieting thoughts that may still be on our mind. We remember the feeling we had as children, free of the everyday realities, responsibilities, and burdens that tend to wear us down as adults. As you spend this time meditating on what matters most in your life, feel a deep and abiding sense of acceptance, warmth, and well-being spread through you. You are at peace with yourself, forgiving of others, at one with the universe.*

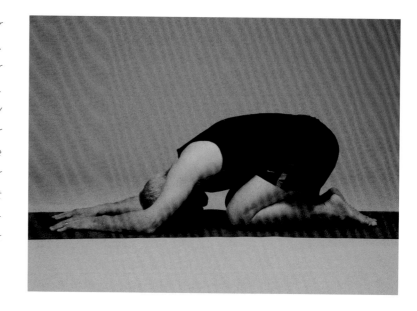

DIRECTIONS

From Table Pose, move your buttocks toward your heels and your head toward the earth and extend your arms forward as you fold into Child's Pose (*top right*). If your head doesn't comfortably reach the floor, rest your forehead on your stacked fists or the backs of your hands (*facing page, top*). If your head easily touches the floor, you may enjoy resting your arms at your sides, palms up (*bottom right*). Feel free to spread your thighs apart if that makes this posture more comfortable. If you have any knee pain, flip the pose upside down, by lying on your back and hugging your knees in toward your chest. Stay here for several breaths, feeling the movement of breath in the back of your body. Child's Pose is a resting posture, so allow each inhalation to fill your body

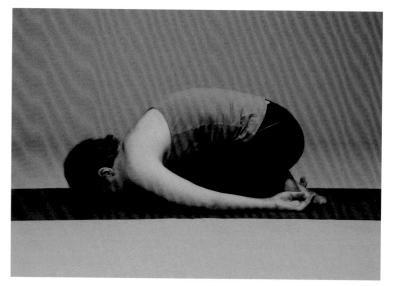

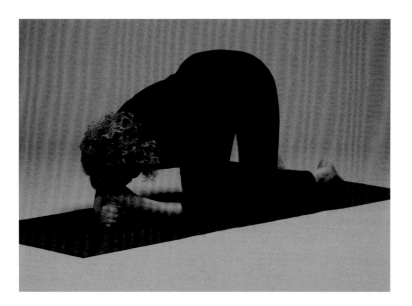

with breath and each exhalation to be an opportunity to relax, release, and let go of any physical and emotional tension, distracting thoughts, or stresses that may still be lingering in your spirit.

ADVANCED TRACK: *Come into Downward-Facing Dog Pose and rest your forehead on a yoga block, if you have one, for a more active resting pose.*

CHAIR MODIFICATION: *Place your chair in front of a bookcase or second chair. Stack your arms to make a pillow for your forehead, and rest them on the bookcase or chair back, letting your head and upper body rest in this support* (bottom left).

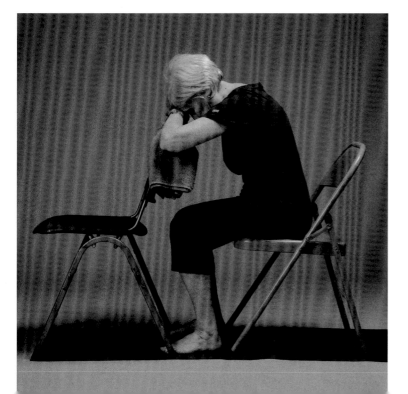

QUESTION

What things bring you a sense of serenity and peace?

YOGA CONNECTION: CHILD'S POSE

Most people find *Balasana*, or Child's Pose, to be an extremely relaxing forward bend. After all, the shape is similar to the fetal position, which is associated with comfort and protection. Since Child's Pose stretches out the lower back, it is often used as a counter-pose after doing back-bending postures. Having the head supported by the floor or on stacked palms or fists allows the neck to relax and release. Common variations include Extended Child's Pose, with the arms stretched forward, and a Wide-Legged Child's Pose for those with round bodies.

KAVANAH

The sound of ocean waves
Waterfalls cascading
The patter of raindrops
Warm wind caressing your face
The sunset over the water
A healthy breakfast
Cool water to drink
Yoga on the beach

Relaxing music
A warm blanket
A roaring fire
A good book
Time to yourself to think
These bring comfort
Serenity and peace
Shalom

PERSONAL KAVANAH

_____

_____

_____

_____

Part IV

Concluding Prayers

12

FINDING BALANCE: *Aleinu* ✦ MUSIC: "Rejoyce" by Jeff Order

לִפְנֵי מֶלֶךְ מַלְכֵי הַמְּלָכִים הַקָּדוֹשׁ בָּרוּךְ הוּא.

Lifnei Melech mal'chei hamlachim HaKadosh Baruch Hu.

Before you, angels of peace, God's spirit is blessed.

Aleinu is the first in the series of concluding prayers in our service. It is traditionally chanted standing, facing the ark or eastward toward Jerusalem. The prayer praises *Adonai* for setting us apart from the other families of the earth, giving us a unique destiny among the nations. In this way we work in partnership with God to perfect our world. Bending and bowing is customary during the *Vaanachnu* portion of the prayer, bending our knees on the word *kor'im*, bowing from the waist on *umishtachavim*, and standing upright on *lifnei Melech*. We perform this choreography in grateful acknowledgment of our humility before the Holy One and in gratitude for our unique place within humanity.

The *Aleinu* prayer *is an expression of our hope for a more perfect world and the unique place of the Jewish people in it. Considering our role and our individual niche in the world, our perspective shifts inward. We rejoice in the blessings of body, mind, creativity, motivation, inspiration, and awareness of spirit that we have been granted. In this Tree Pose balance, we establish our firm connection with the earth, sending roots down first through one leg, then another, getting grounded as we bring ourselves into balance on one leg. We are inspired by the diversity of uniquely beautiful trees in nature and we seek balance, with the intention of allowing our posture to represent our individuality and the unique qualities we possess. Letting go of judgments and self-criticism, we recognize that our courage and strength will provide the stability necessary to balance the many aspects of our lives so that we can blossom into the divine spark that exists within us. In this way, we can fulfill the intention of this prayer, to bring our world into harmony.*

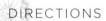

DIRECTIONS

Standing tall in Mountain Pose, inhale while extending your arms out to the sides at shoulder height, then exhale and relax your shoulders down away from your ears. (Feel free to lightly touch a wall for support if you like.) Root down through your left foot as you pick up your right heel, turn your right knee out forty-five degrees, and slide the sole of your right foot against your left ankle (*right*). For more challenge, pick up your right foot and place the sole along the inside of your left leg, either above or below your knee (*facing page, left*). Anchor your gaze at a spot on the horizon to steady your balance. If you feel balanced, extend your arms into any position that expresses your own "inner tree." Lengthen your body up through the crown of your head as you root down through your left foot, and balance for several breaths. Return to Mountain Pose and repeat on the other side.

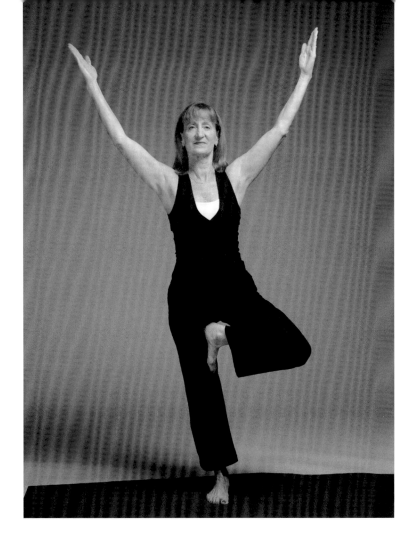

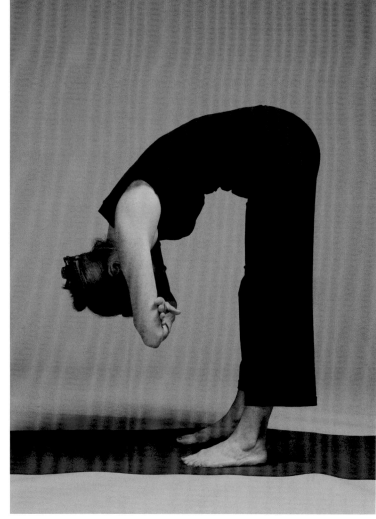

ADVANCED TRACK: *Bring your heel into the little notch at the top of the thigh, and look skyward as you bring your hands into Temple Mudra with your upper arms close to your ears. Breathe and balance. Bring both feet to the floor, hinge from the waist into full forward bend, and grasp your elbows (above right). Rock from side to side. Hinging up, bring your arms up over your head, then open them out into a "Y" position—called Hallelujah Arms—and swing them from side to side gently. Finish by bringing your palms together at your heart.*

CHAIR MODIFICATION: *Sit toward the front of your chair with both feet firmly on the ground. Then lift your right heel up, turn the toes of the right foot out forty-five degrees, and slide your right heel against the inside of your left leg (appendix, fig. 12.1). Extend your arms out to the sides at shoulder height. This may be enough sensation, but if you want more challenge, float the toes of your right foot off the floor.*

YOGA CONNECTION: FINDING BALANCE

Balance poses teach some of yoga's most important lessons: getting grounded, finding your center, staying focused, maintaining concentration, and steadying the mind. The process of learning to balance—with its inevitable falling and trying again—cultivates patience and persistence, humility and good humor. These qualities help us do more than stay balanced in yoga postures. They help us stay balanced in life.

QUESTION

What quality about yourself is unique? What kind of tree matches your personality and nature?

KAVANAH

I am strong as a mighty oak
I am flexible as a weeping willow
I am beautiful as a cherry tree in bloom
I am prickly as a cactus
I am flirty as a palm

I am round as a linden tree
I am reflective like the leaves of an aspen
I am humbled and bow low like a Joshua tree
I am sappy as the pine
I am wise like the ancient redwood

PERSONAL KAVANAH

_____

_____

_____

_____

13

REMEMBER: *Kaddish* ◆ MUSIC: "The Rest of Faith" by Ira Fein

עֹשֶׂה שָׁלוֹם בִּמְרוֹמָיו הוּא יַעֲשֶׂה שָׁלוֹם
עָלֵינוּ וְעַל כָּל יִשְׂרָאֵל, וְאִמְרוּ: אָמֵן.

Oseh shalom bimromav hu yaaseh shalom aleinu v'al kol Yisrael, v'imru: Amen.

May the Holy One who makes peace in the heavens
Send peace to all who are bereaved and in need of healing.

Kaddish Yatom, the Mourner's *Kaddish*, is a hymn of praise to God and a prayer for God's presence to be revealed to us on earth. Various forms of *Kaddish* are used to mark the end of each part of the worship service. The custom of reciting the *Kaddish* for a year after the death of a loved one and on the anniversary of that death (called *yahrzeit*) originated in the Rhineland during the Crusades (eleventh century). It is recited at the conclusion of our service, giving mourners the opportunity to remember loved ones who are no longer living and bringing communal acknowledgment and support for loss, grief, and bereavement.

When someone we love dies, *our worlds are turned up-side down. Sometimes it is a struggle to get out of bed, to face the world and move on with our lives. Our body remembers grief and stores it deep within our muscles and joints. We begin to release our pain and disorientation by inverting our bodies, resting our legs up the wall or on a chair, going up into shoulder or head stand if we are experienced and comfortable with these postures. We take a moment to name a loved one whose body has passed into eternity and whose spirit lingers within our heart and mind. We are aware of the blood of life flowing into our heart center, the weight of sadness releasing from the soles of our feet. Our breath carries with it the memories that surge throughout our being as we spend a few moments in remembrance.*

DIRECTIONS

Sit on the floor about a hand's distance away from a wall, with your legs parallel to the wall. Then swing your legs up the wall as you rest your back on the floor (*right*). Feel free to adjust the distance of your buttocks to the wall—they can be flush against the wall or further away—so that your body feels as comfortable as possible with your legs supported by the wall and your body supported by the floor. Allow your arms to rest at your sides, about six to eight inches away from your body, palms up. Close your eyes, and invite your breath to slow and deepen as you rest comfortably in this supported posture.

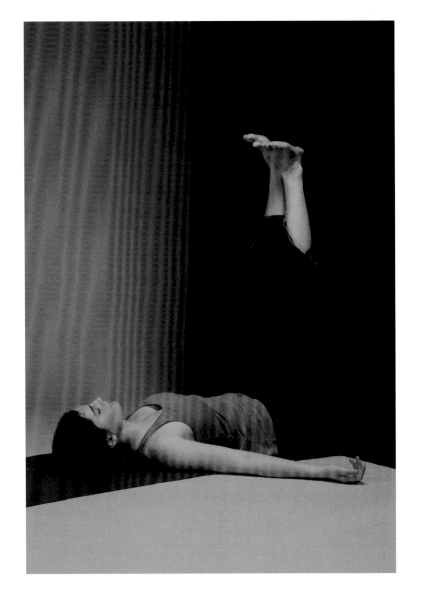

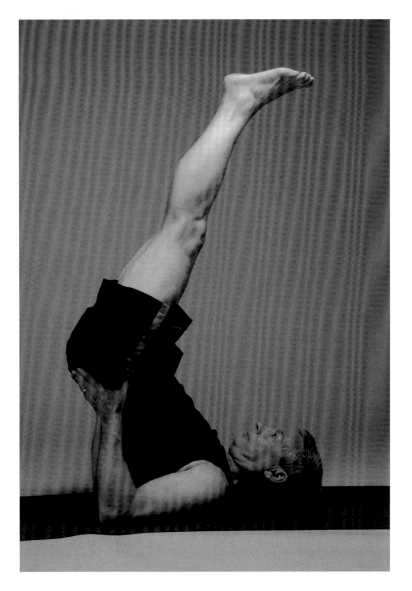

ADVANCED TRACK: *Try another inversion such as shoulder stand. Begin lying on the floor with your knees bent over your chest, arms on the floor palms down. On an exhalation, lift your hips up, and place your hands on your lower back for support. Rest the weight of your hips on your hands, and if you like, straighten your legs (left). When you are ready, roll back down.*

GENTLE VARIATION: *Lie on your back and rest your legs on a chair (appendix, fig. 13.1).*

CHAIR MODIFICATION: *Rest your legs on a chair placed in front of you (appendix, fig. 13.2).*

QUESTION

Whose memory do you carry strongly in your heart? Imagine your grief rising through your feet and releasing from your body.

YOGA CONNECTION: RESTORATIVE POSTURES

Unlike the Western exercise mentality that says the harder you work, the better the results, in yoga we often go deeper by *not* working—by relaxing, releasing, and letting go. In yoga, learning how to "undo" is as important (and for some people *more* important) as learning how to "do." Since yoga is as much about undoing as doing, sometimes the most appropriate and healing practice will involve lying still and focusing on your breath. Restorative postures place the body in a supported position—such as lying down with a bolster under the knees or reclining on a stack of folded blankets—and cultivate the surprisingly difficult practice of totally releasing all muscle tension and surrendering completely to the earth. Legs Up the Wall Pose, also known as *Viparita Karani*, can be particularly restorative for people who are on their feet all day, since it involves inverting the legs—reversing the pull of gravity on the fluids and tissues in the legs.

KAVANAH

In the blink of an eye
Whole world changes
People that we love
Suddenly are gone
All that we have
Is but lent to us
In the blink of an eye
Ashes turn to dust

In the blink of an eye
Our lives flash before us
Thinking of things
That we should have done
Promises made
Promises broken
In the blink of an eye
We feel so alone

We turn to the One
From whom we draw comfort
When family and friends
Aren't enough
We look for the strength
From deep inside us
The spirit of our loved one
Forever in our hearts

PERSONAL KAVANAH

_____

_____

_____

14

LETTING GO: *Adon Olam* ✦ MUSIC: "Only at the Ocean Ver. I" by Steve Povlo

בְּיָדוֹ אַפְקִיד רוּחִי, בְּעֵת אִישַׁן וְאָעִירָה.
וְעִם רוּחִי גְּוִיָּתִי, יְיָ לִי וְלֹא אִירָא.

B'yado afkid ruchi, b'eit ishan v'a-irah.
V'im ruchi g'viyati, Adonai li v'lo ira.

Into Your hands I entrust my spirit, when I sleep and when I wake.
And with body and spirit the Holy One is with me, I shall not fear.

Adon Olam is a strophic hymn that is often sung at the end of a worship service. The final verse of *Adon Olam* quoted here leads us to believe that the poem may have been meant to be recited before bedtime with the *Sh'ma*, or at the end of life. The verse has become part of contemporary healing practices, as it invokes the image of entrusting our spirits to God's care. The numerous melodies that exist to accompany these words attest to their power and ability to connect us with the healing power of the Divine.

We conclude our service *with a series of releasing, relaxing, and healing prayers. These represent the ultimate goal of our yoga worship today: to internalize what our bodies have experienced, to memorize what our spirits have told us, and to free our minds of any lingering negative feelings or worrisome thoughts. This is your time for relinquishing control, of letting go. It is time to relax and release any unwanted physical and emotional tensions by stretching your muscles thoroughly. Your muscles and joints are archives of past experiences and may store pain, fear, and other negative emotions deep within their protective layers. Pay attention to your body and your breath as you stretch. With each inhalation and with each exhalation, send your body the intention of releasing any unnecessary physical or emotional pain, lingering negative feelings, or worrisome thoughts. As your stretching exposes hidden emotions, you may feel the need to cry or sigh or breathe more deeply to completely free your muscles and release.*

DIRECTIONS

Lie on your back with your knees bent and your feet flat on the floor. Take each stretch just to the point of mild tension, then use your breath to help you soften and release, perhaps taking you deeper into the pose. With each stretch you may feel some discomfort, which can be an inherent part of the growth process—you learn how to breathe through uncomfortable sensations until your body finds ease. If you experience pain, however, be sure to back off. Allow your body to retreat just a bit, to a place that is comfortable yet challenging, where you feel a sensation of stretch that is not hurtful or a strain. Bring your right thigh to your chest and extend your right heel into the air. You may want to deepen the stretch by gently placing your hands behind your thigh or your calf and drawing your leg toward you (*facing page, top*). Draw circles in the air with your toes, enlivening your ankles. Point and flex your foot, feeling the effect on the muscles in the back of your leg (*appendix, fig. 14.1*). Now bend your knee and bring your right ankle to your left thigh, just below the knee. This may be enough sensation, but if you're ready for more, reach your hands forward, pick up your left foot, and hug your left thigh into Keyhole Pose (*facing page, bottom left*). Invite your breath to help soften any places that feel the sensation of stretch. Then bring both feet back to the ground, knees bent, and take a moment to notice how you feel—and any differences between the right and left leg. Repeat this series of stretches by extending the left leg up, stretching, rotating the foot, pointing and flexing, and concluding by placing the left ankle on the right thigh and hugging it to release the right hip. Now extend both feet up toward the ceiling and straighten both legs, feeling a deep stretch in both legs. Then bend both knees and bring them out to the sides, showing the soles of the feet toward the sky. Hold your thighs, your legs, or the soles of your feet. This is Happy Baby Pose (*facing page, bottom right*). Rock from side to side, releasing the hips and muscles supporting the spine. Now bring the soles of your feet together and release your legs to the earth, knees extending out to the sides in Cobbler's Pose. Extend your arms up over your head and release. When you are ready, bring your knees together, the soles of your feet to the floor, and your arms out into "T" posi-

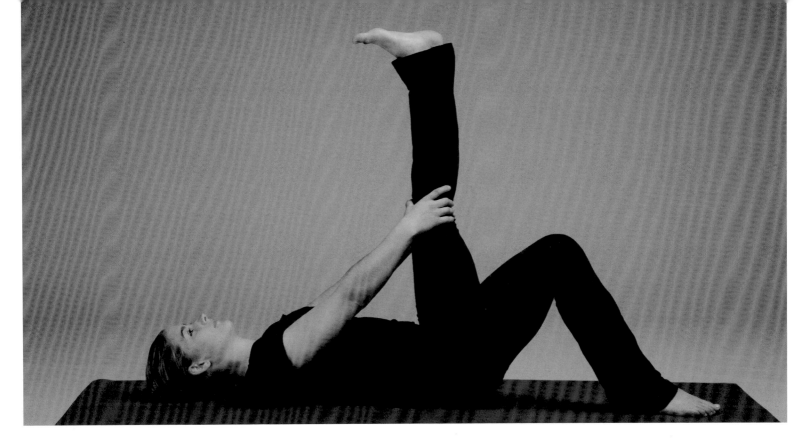

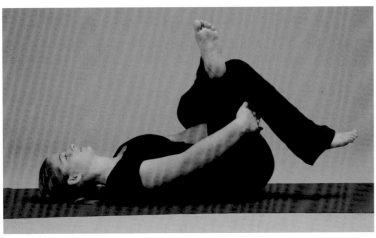

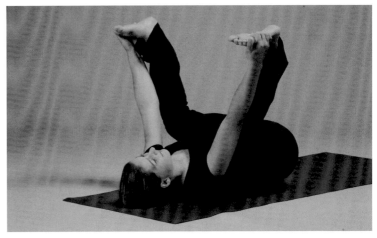

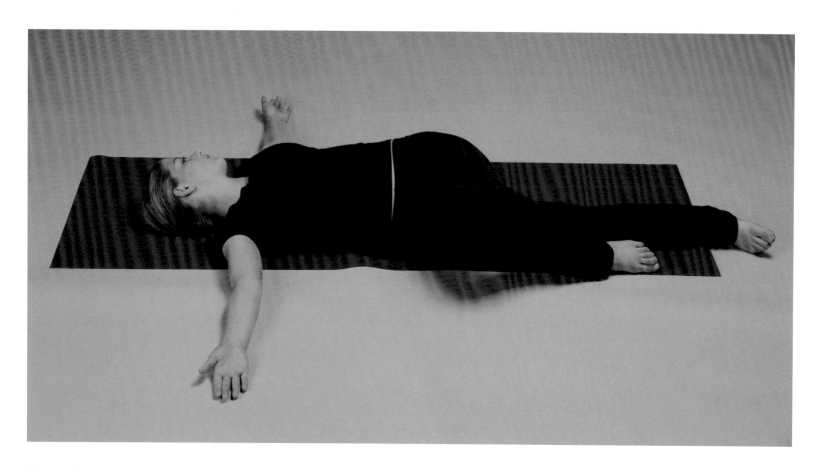

tion at shoulder height. Then exhale as you drop both knees to the right and look to the left (*above*). Stay here for a few breaths, then inhale while moving back to the center, then exhale as you drop both knees to the left and look to the right. Rest here for a few breaths, then inhale while moving back to the center, and hug both knees in to your chest, gently rocking from side to side, relaxing the muscles in your lower back.

ADVANCED TRACK: *Hold your big toes during the leg stretch. Variation: Sitting leg stretches with legs extended out in front, then out to the sides in a "V" shape.*

CHAIR MODIFICATION: *Sitting tall in your chair, slide your right foot forward, and flex and point your right foot, keeping your breath flowing (facing page, left). Make circles with the toes, energizing the ankles.*

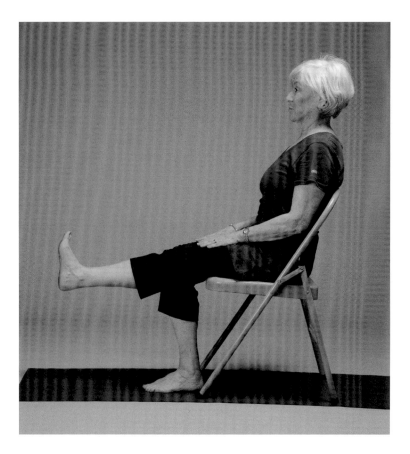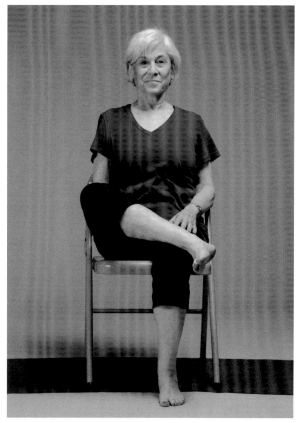

Then inhale as you straighten your right leg out in front of you, and exhale while moving it back down. Continue a few times, moving with your breath, then repeat with the left leg. If you can, rest your right ankle on your left thigh or left shin, then flex and point the foot and make ankle circles (top right). On an inhalation, spread the toes of your right foot out so that no toe touches another toe; then on an exhalation, clench the toes in a "fist." Repeat, moving with your breath. Repeat this sequence with the opposite leg.

QUESTION

Is there a painful experience or memory you feel released from as you stretch? Continue to send your breath to anywhere that feels tight or needs to open and release.

YOGA CONNECTION: GOING DEEPER

The ancient texts on yoga tell us that a posture should be "steady and comfortable" or, according to some translations, "relaxed and stable" or "sweet and calm." So it is essential to *avoid strain in any pose*. The yogic approach is to take your movement to the place where you feel a sensation of mild tension, then stay there and breathe—perhaps going deeper by relaxing into the stretch, rather than by muscling your way into it. Just as you can't force a rosebud to open, pushing yourself into a posture can lead to injury. Instead, allow your pose to deepen with the tools of patience, gravity, and your breath. With time and practice, your posture will blossom and grow.

KAVANAH

O High and Hidden One
Give me a window
To see what is hiding
Deep in my body's memory
Like a kaleidoscope
Of colors
I see and release

As I breathe and stretch
Opening and discovering
Peeling away the layers
Fathoming my ability
To relinquish
What is binding me
I am free

PERSONAL KAVANAH

_____

_____

_____

_____

15

SURRENDER: Priestly Benediction ✦ MUSIC: "Bija" by Todd Norian

יְבָרֶכְךָ יְיָ וְיִשְׁמְרֶךָ. יָאֵר יְיָ פָּנָיו אֵלֶיךָ וִיחֻנֶּךָּ.
יִשָּׂא יְיָ פָּנָיו אֵלֶיךָ וְיָשֵׂם לְךָ שָׁלוֹם.

Y'varech'cha Adonai v'yishm'recha. Ya-eir Adonai panav eilecha vichuneka.
Yisa Adonai panav eilecha v'yaseim l'cha shalom.

May the Holy One bless you and nurture you. May the Holy One shine through you and inspire you.
May the Holy One bring you a sense of well-being, wholeness, and peace.

Continuing the concluding part of our worship, we give our bodies time to release and restore, to relax and memorize all that we have experienced through our worship and yoga practice. The Priestly Benediction, taken from *Parashat Naso*, Numbers 6:24–26, is recited at times of blessing such as weddings and other life-cycle events, these words were bestowed upon Moses as he passed the yoke of leadership to his brother Aaron before his death. The blessing has become synonymous with healing and our own ability to receive as well as bestow blessing and to share our hope for restoration and healing with the world.

Our final embodiment *is a blessing of rest and renewal for ourselves, a time to surrender, relax, and absorb the full realization of our prayer practice today. Sometimes the hardest pose is to be still, inviting ourselves to completely let go and sink into deep and profound rest. Take a moment to say thank you to your feet for bringing you to your mat, your* mishkan, *your holy place. Thank your hands for helping you do God's work in the world. Acknowledge the fullness of your heart, opened and filled with holiness and blessing. Say thank-you to your mind for enabling you to reason, question, and interpret all that your body has revealed to you today. Know that you can call upon the personal* kavanah, *the intention you created for yourself today, whenever and wherever you should need strength and support. Feel blessed with every fiber of your being as you imagine the child within you being totally cared for, nurtured, supported, and loved.*

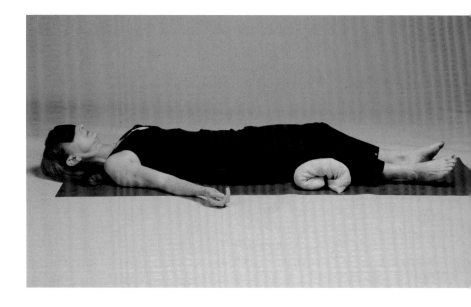

DIRECTIONS

Feel free to put your socks on, cover yourself with a sweater or blanket, turn off the lights, and let yourself sink onto your mat with your hands out to your sides, palms facing up and your legs stretched out comfortably in front of you, ankles splayed comfortably outward (*above and facing page*). If you experience any back discomfort, feel free to bend your knees or place a rolled mat or towel under you knees. Imagine your mat is a comfortable bed. Invite your breath to slow and deepen, so that with each ex-

halation more and more of your body weight releases down into the support of the bed. Picture a blanket being drawn up over your body, beginning with your feet, up over your legs, abdomen, and chest, then tucked up under your chin. You are completely surrounded by warmth and protection, a cocoon of relaxation. Bring your attention to your face and allow all the muscles of expression to soften and relax. Let your eyes rest back in their sockets. Release the hinge of your jaw so that your teeth gently part, and allow your tongue to fall away from the roof of your mouth. Let your head become heavy, dropping into the earth so that your neck and shoulders are free of their weight. Soften your throat and relax your arms, wrists, hands, fingers, and thumbs. Bring your attention to your internal organs. Sense the steady beating of your heart, and take a moment to give blessing for

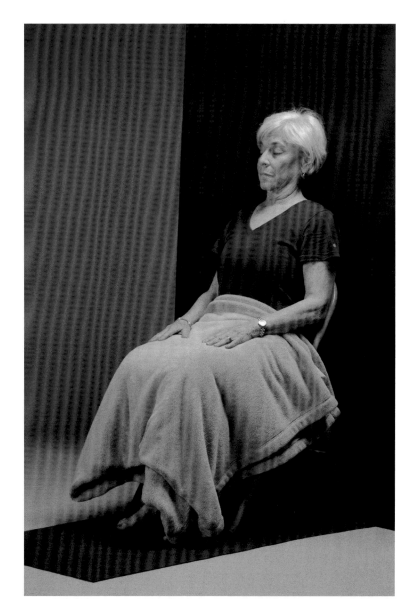

the openings in your body and the life-giving blood that flows to your organs through veins and arteries: *n'kavim, n'kavim, chalulim, chalulim*, the opening and closings we extol in our prayer *Asher Yatzar*. Were one of them to fail, we know that our bodies could not function. Relax your hips and your thighs, and release your legs, feet, and toes. Invite your bones to become heavy, so that their weight drops toward the earth, and allow your flesh to soften away from the bones. Invite the skin all over your body to soften and release. Trust the floor to hold you up. Trust that everything is as it should be. For the next few minutes, do nothing but relax, release, and surrender completely to the earth.

When you are ready, bring your awareness back to the room, and gently begin to move your fingers and toes. See if you can stay connected to the sense of stillness and peace that you've realized through your practice. See if, as you return to your day, you can revisit this sense of peace and share it with others. At your own time, bend your knees and roll onto your side, creating a pillow with your arms. Rest for a few moments before you bring yourself to sitting.

Question

How can you share the sense of peace and stillness you experienced in *Yoga Shalom* with others? Take your practice with you into your day.

YOGA CONNECTION: CORPSE POSE

This yogic practice, called *Savasana*, or Corpse Pose, is a head-to-toe tension reliever that cultivates a sense of deep relaxation. While it looks pretty simple, since, after all, you're lying still and doing nothing, it's actually among the most difficult poses to master because it requires *totally* letting go of all physical tension, quieting the mind, and surrendering completely to the earth. Practicing active postures first helps release tension and enhance the flow of energy throughout the body, so that when you finally come to rest in Corpse Pose, your body and mind can come into stillness and connect with the still, small voice of the heart.

KAVANAH

With each breath
I expand my ability
To relax myself
In any situation.
I can bring my awareness inward
To recall the feelings
I experience on my mat.
When I am angry
When I am frustrated

When I am feeling lost
I breathe,
And with each full breath
I feel quiet stillness returning
Calmness overtaking me
Stress melting away
My inner sight refocusing.
With each inhale,
And exhale,
I am restored.

PERSONAL KAVANAH

_____

_____

_____

_____

16

בָּרוּךְ אַתָּה יְיָ רוֹפֵא הַחוֹלִים.

Baruch atah, Adonai, rofei hacholim.

Blessed are You, **Adonai,** *who brings wholeness and healing.*

Mi Shebeirach means "One who blesses" and is the prayer for healing. Traditionally this prayer is recited during the Torah service at the conclusion of the *aliyot,* or reading of the weekly *parashah* (portion). With the popularity of Debbie Friedman's now legendary melody, the prayer has become a regular part of many worship practices and continues to be sung at the most painful times in our lives.

We complete our practice *today with the* Mi Shebeirach *prayer by channeling our thoughts and energy to those in need of healing of the mind, healing of the body, and healing of the spirit. Coping with illness can be one of the most difficult challenges in life. Whether it be the illness of a parent, sibling, child, friend, or ourself, working through the emotions and pain associated with the everyday stresses of illness can leave us weak, depressed, drained, and depleted. Through breathing, yoga, prayer, and meditation, we visualize ourselves moving past the most difficult moments in our lives to a bright and positive future.*

We close into a circle as we encircle our arms around one another, mirroring the circle of the planet, the circle of life, the circle of faith. We call upon the energy we feel flowing around the circle, the power we feel surrounding us as our prayers draw together in a call for strength, unity, and courage. If you are practicing alone on your mat today, bring your hands into Prayer Pose at heart center, and close your eyes. Visualize healing as you call upon a deep and abiding hope and belief that your prayers make a difference. Send your healing intention to those in pain and to those who minister to those who are ill. Extend your healing prayers to those suffering on our planet and around the world. Take a moment to name someone, either aloud or in your heart, who is in need of healing.

DIRECTIONS

Stand in a circle, and place your arms around those around you (*facing page*). Or, sit comfortably on your mat with your hands at your heart center.

YOGIC CONNECTION: HEALING YOGA

Although yoga practices are designed to enhance our well-being, yogic tradition does not view improved health as an end in itself but rather as a quality necessary to properly connect with the spirit. The ancient yogis considered disease to be an obstacle to enlightenment. After all, it's difficult to sit still in meditation and unite with the Divine if you have a pounding headache or a stomachache. Likewise, if illness or sedentary habits have left you too weak and inflexible to sit comfortably, yoga postures and breathing practices can help you become healthy and strong enough to sit quietly and meditate. The body is considered a temple of the soul, and yoga practice helps maintain this precious vessel.

QUESTION

Who is in need of your healing prayers? It can be yourself, or someone else, or the world. Feel the energy and life force of healing moving throughout the healing circle and reaching whoever is in need.

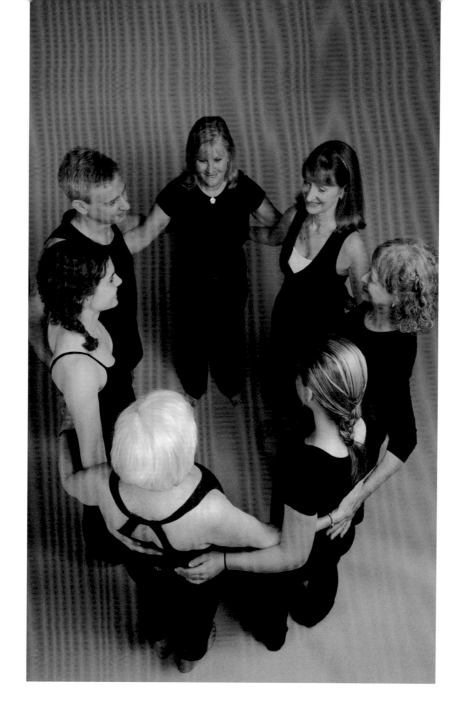

KAVANAH

Mi shebeirach Avoteinu
Avraham, Yitzchak v'Yaakov
Mi shebeirach Imoteinu
Sarah, Rivkah, Leah v'Rachel.
May the One who blessed our Mothers
May the One who blessed our Fathers
Hear our prayer and bless us as well.
Bless us with the power of Your healing

Bless us with the power of Your hope
May our hearts be filled with understanding
And strengthened by the power of Your love
Bless us with the vision for tomorrow
Help us to reach out to those in pain
May the warmth of friendship ease our sorrow
Give us courage, give us faith
Show us the way!

PERSONAL KAVANAH

_____

_____

_____

_____

CONCLUSION

+ Be kind to yourself, move slowly, and take your time as you make the transition back into your regular day.

+ Remember that you have the ability to bring yourself back to your practice and the *kavanah*, or intention, you created for yourself at any time should you feel stressed. Simply close your eyes for a moment, take a few deep breaths, and release any anxiety you may be feeling.

+ You may want to drink plenty of water throughout the day to cleanse and replenish.

+ Repeat this practice as often as possible. Regular practice will give you the confidence to move away from the DVD and use the book and CD to create your own unique practice.

APPENDIX

CHAPTER 1:
BREATHING AND CENTERING

CHAPTER 2:
RESTORATION OF THE SOUL

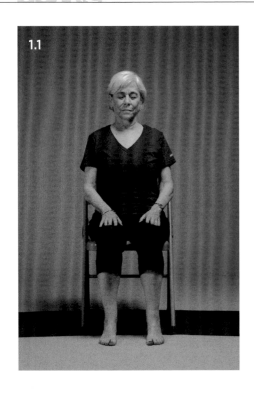

1.1

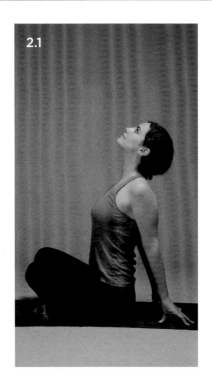

2.1

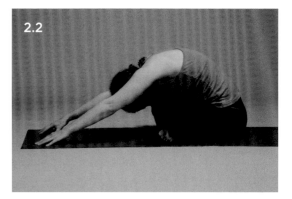

2.2

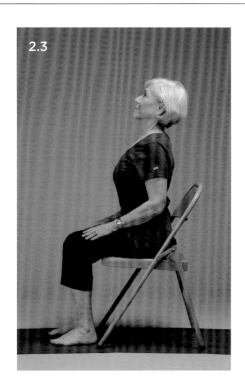
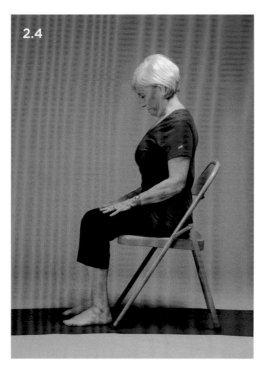
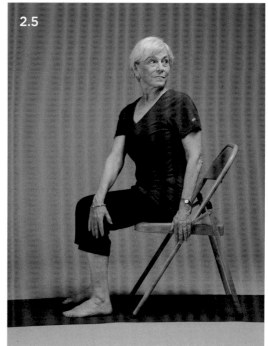

2.3

2.4

2.5

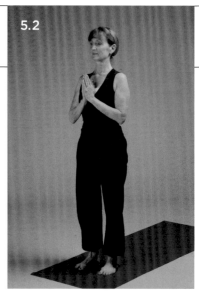

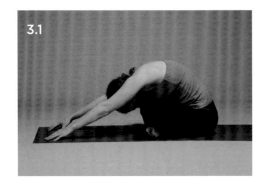

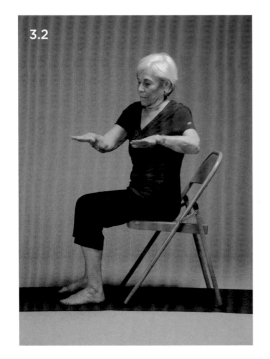

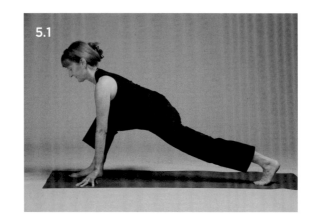

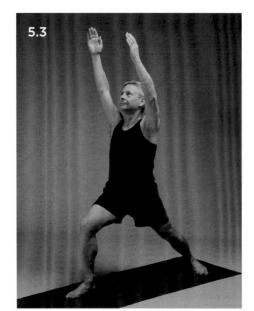

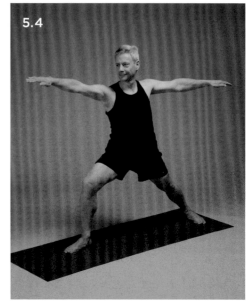

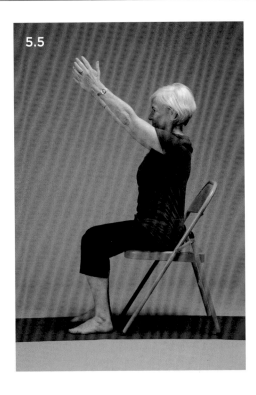

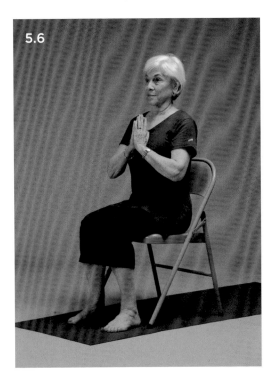

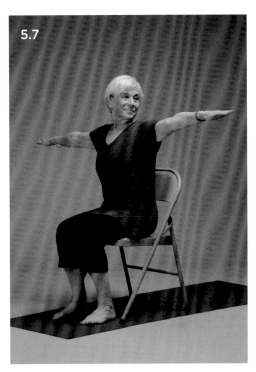

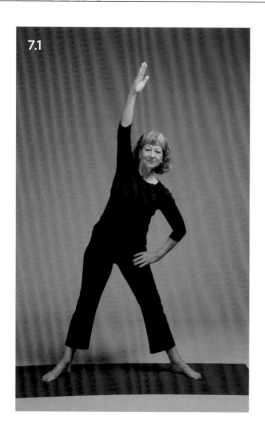

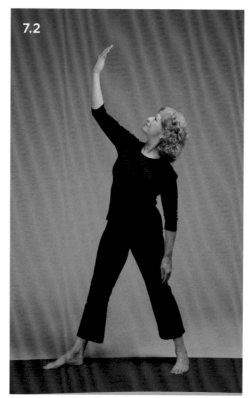

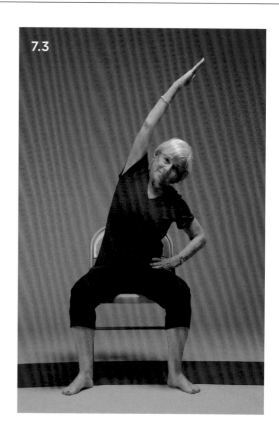

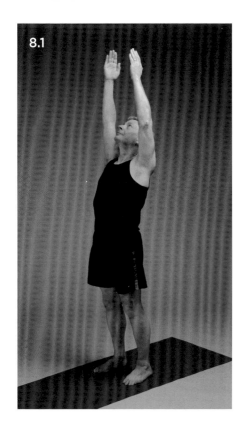

8.1

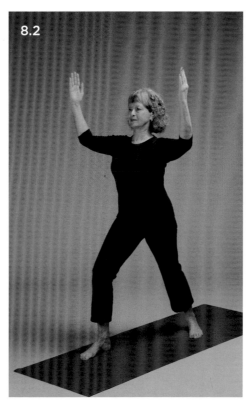

8.2

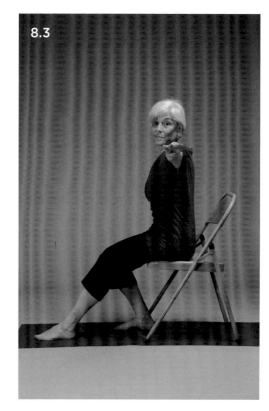

8.3

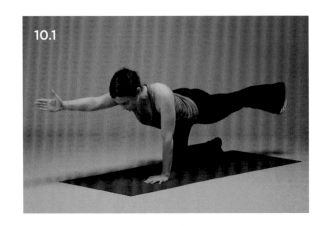

10.1

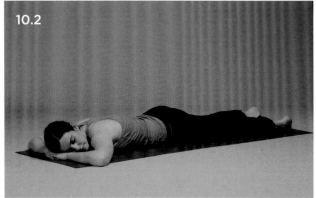

10.2

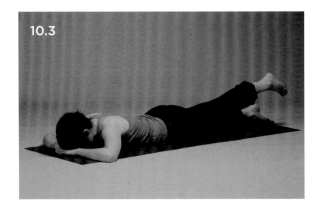

10.3

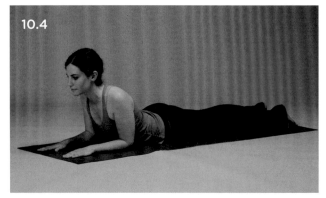

10.4

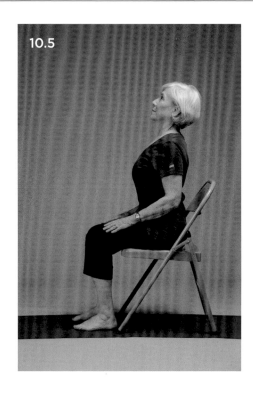

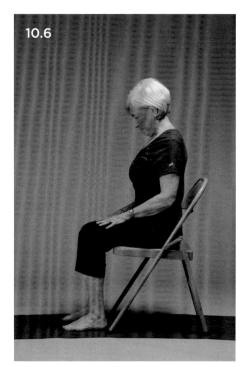

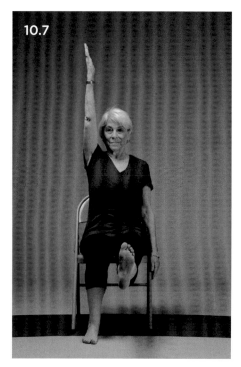

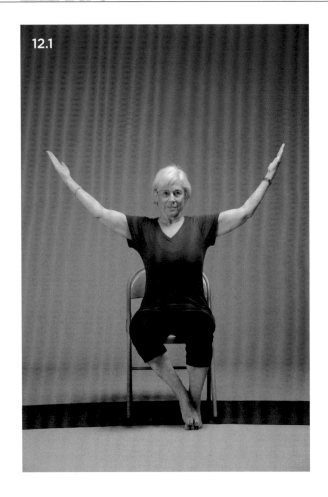

12.1

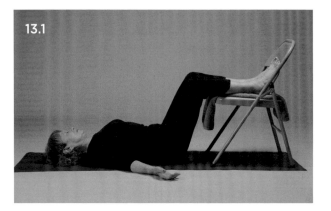

13.1

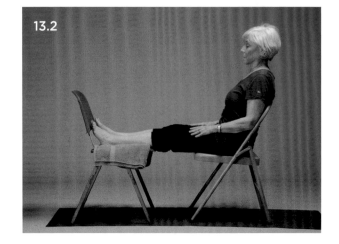

13.2

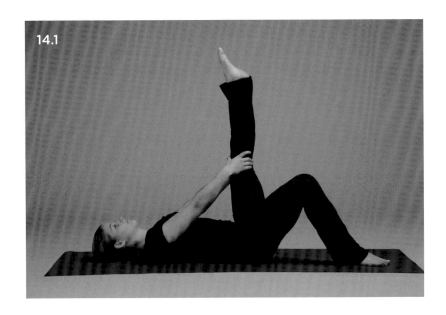

14.1

ACKNOWLEDGMENTS

This book would not have come to fruition without the help and encouragement from many special people. First and foremost, I would like to thank my yoga teachers, Kay Sipple of Leawood, Kansas, and Alicia Cuervo of Yin Yang Yoga in Olney, Maryland, whose teaching, wisdom, and guidance have helped me in my practice of yoga and encouraged me on my journey. Thank you to Rabbi Susie Moskowitz, who first embarked upon this adventure with me at our first yoga worship service at the URJ Biennial in Minneapolis. Thanks to the staff of the Union for Reform Judaism, especially Cantor Alane Katzew, for giving me the opportunity to explore the idea of yoga and worship by extending me the invitations to lead *Yoga Shalom* that led to this book. Thanks to Rabbi Steven Fox, whose words of wisdom brought me insight. Many thanks to Rabbi Hara Person, who first saw the book proposal and thought it had promise and potential. Thank you to Michael Goldberg, who has shepherded and patiently focused us on what the book needed to contain and worked with us in completing it, and the other members of the URJ Books and Music staff who have contributed to the book: Victor Ney, Stephen Becker, Steve Brodsky, Jessica Katz, Jonathan Levine, Rebecca Rosenfeld, and Michael Silber. Thank you to Jimmy and Sue Klau, who brought me to be an artist-in-residence at Temple Beth Shalom in San Juan and offered me the hospitality that gave me the time and tranquility to write much of the book. Thank you to Rabbi John Friedman and Judea Reform Congregation in Durham, North Carolina, for extending their hospitality for the DVD recording. Thank you to Robin Dinerman, Margie Satinsky, Howie Shareff, Edward Skloot, Michal Unna, and Eleanor Ostrinsky for participating in the DVD recording. Thanks Rabbi Michael Feshbach and Susan Zemsky, the leadership, and members of Temple Shalom in Chevy Chase, Maryland, my spiritual home and community, for their continued support. Thank you to the many participants in *Yoga Shalom* workshops over the years whose feedback and generosity of spirit have contributed to the final version of this worship practice.

A special thank you to Carol Krucoff, whose vision and belief in this practice culminated in the publishing of this book. Without Carol's experience, knowledge, and understanding of yoga, guidance, and editing, this book could not have been created.

Many thanks to my family, my husband, Andy, and my children, Emily and Louis, for their love and support during the long hours of practice, writing, recording, and travel. I would like to thank and acknowledge the support of my parents, Marvin Lipco *z"l* and Shirley Lipco Baker, whose love and encouragement over my lifetime have given me the self-confidence to believe that anything is possible with hard work and perseverance. Finally, thank you to "my rabbi," Rabbi Arthur Kolatch, *z"l*, who taught me that blessings from without come from what you have within. Each of us has those blessings to share, and I hope this book empowers that light within us to shine forth.

Lisa Levine

I'm grateful to the many yoga teachers I've studied with over the years, in particular to my mentor Esther Myers, may her memory be for a blessing. I continually learn from my yoga students and yoga therapy clients and offer them sincere thanks for allowing me the gift of service. Immeasurable thanks to my family, my husband, Mitchell, son Max, and daughter Rae, for their love and support. Thanks to the students who participated in this DVD: Edward Skloot, Margie Satinsky, Michal Unna, Howie Shareff, and Robin Dinerman, plus a special hug of gratitude to my remarkable mother, Eleanor Ostrinsky, "the lady in the chair," who is—and has always been—smarter than the average mommy. Thanks, too, to my cool cousin Kenny Weinstein for modeling the poses so expertly in this book. Heartfelt thanks to our rabbis, John Friedman and Leah Berkowitz, for allowing us to use our beautiful synagogue as a setting for the DVD. And deep appreciation to Cantor Lisa Levine, whose vision, artistry, and beautiful voice have created an extraordinary vehicle for Jewish worship.

Carol Krucoff

We dedicate this book to our friend, teacher, and mentor Debbie Friedman, *z"l*, whose spirit and vision for healing and renewal gave birth to an entire movement of self-realization and deep reflection for health and well-being.

CREDITS

BOOK DESIGN AND COMPOSITION: Judith Stagnitto Abbate/
Abbate Design/www.abbatedesign.com
COVER DESIGN: Michael J. Silber

PHOTOGRAPHY: Carl Caruso
MODELS: Diana Dinerman, Robin Dinerman, Rachel Friedman,
Carol Krucoff, Lisa Levine, Beryl Tretter, Kenneth Weinstein

DVD RECORDED at Judea Reform Congregation, Durham, NC
DVD PRODUCED by David Hardy
AUDIO by David Hardy
CAST: Robin Dinerman, Carol Krucoff, Lisa Levine, Eleanor
Ostrinsky, Margie Satinsky, Howie Shareff, Edward Skloot,
Michal Unna

CD RECORDED, MIXED, AND MASTERED by Dave Vergauen at Order
Productions, Baltimore, MD
VOCALS AND GUITAR: Lisa Levine
PERCUSSION: Mark Suresh Schlanger
CELLO: Diane Cline

ADDITIONAL MUSIC CREDITS

1. Flute Stream (Ira Fein)
Performed by Ira Fein, from the CD *Come Beloved*
Music by Ira Fein
© 2005 Ira Fein
www.healingmusic.org/hmo/IraFein

2. Breathe (Terry Lieberstein)
Performed by Terry Lieberstein, from the CD *Center of the Storm*
Music and lyrics by Terry Lieberstein
© 2001 Lovingstone Productions
www.lovingstone.com

3. Elohai N'shama (Shefa Gold)
Performed by Cantor Lisa Levine
Music by Rabbi Shefa Gold, Hebrew text from liturgy; additional
music and English lyrics by Lisa Levine
© 1989 C-DEEP
www.rabbishefagold.com

4. Nishmat Kol Chai (Lisa Levine)
Performed by Cantor Lisa Levine
Music and English lyrics by Lisa Levine, Hebrew text from liturgy
© 2001 L & M Productions (ASCAP)

5. Bar'chu (Craig Taubman)
Performed by Craig Taubman, from the CD *Friday Night Live*
Music by Craig Taubman, Hebrew text from liturgy
© 1999 Sweet Louise Music (BMI)
www.craignco.com

6. Yotzeir Or (Traditional)
Performed by Cantor Lisa Levine
Folk melody, Hebrew text from liturgy, additional English lyrics by Lisa Levine

7. Open Up Our Eyes (Jeff Klepper)
Performed by Cantor Lisa Levine
Music and lyrics by Jeff Klepper, based on liturgy
© 1997 Jeff Klepper
www.jeffklepper.com

8. Listen (Ira Fein)
Performed by Ira Fein, from the CD *Come Beloved*
Music by Ira Fein
© 2005 Ira Fein
www.healingmusic.org/hmo/IraFein

9. Mi Chamocha (Bonia Shur)
Performed by Cantor Lisa Levine
Music by Bonia Shur, Hebrew text from Exodus 15:11
© 1997 Bonia Shur
"Tzur Yisrael" based on nusach, adapted by Lisa Levine

10. Adonai S'fatai (Traditional)
Performed by Cantor Lisa Levine
Music traditional, Hebrew text from Psalm 51:17, "Halleluyah" descant music by Lisa Levine

11. HaMakom (YofiYah)
Performed by YofiYah, from the CD *Kabbalah Kirtan*
Music by YofiYah, Hebrew text based on Genesis 28:17
© 2005 YofiYah
www.soundstrue.com

12. Elohai N'tzor (Danny Maseng)
Performed by Danny Maseng, from the CD *Soul on Fire*
Music by Danny Maseng, Hebrew text from liturgy
© 2000 Danny Maseng
www.dannymaseng.com

13. Rejoyce (Jeff Order)
Performed by Jeff Order, from the CD *Sea of Tranquility*
Music by Jeff Order; "Lifnei Melech" music by Lisa Levine, Hebrew text from liturgy
© 1989 Order Productions
www.orderproductions.com

14. The Rest of Faith (Ira Fein)
Performed by Ira Fein, from the CD *Come Beloved*
Music by Ira Fein
© 2005 Ira Fein
www.healingmusic.org/hmo/IraFein

15. Only at the Ocean Ver. I (Steve Povlo)
Performed by Steve Povlo, from the CD *Music for the Mind*
Music by Steve Povlo
© 2006 Steve Povlo
www.myspace.com/povlo

16. Bija (Todd Norian)
Performed by Todd Norian, from the CD *Bija: Soothing Music and Mantras for Yoga and Meditation*
Music by Todd Norian
© 2003 Todd Norian
www.deeppeaceyoga.com

17. Hear Our Prayer (Lisa Levine)
Performed by Cantor Lisa Levine, previously unreleased
Music and English lyrics by Lisa Levine, Hebrew text based on liturgy
© 2008 L & M Productions (ASCAP)
www.cantorlisalevine.com

ABOUT THE AUTHORS

CANTOR LISA LEVINE serves as cantor of Temple Shalom in Chevy Chase, Maryland. She earned a bachelor's degree in music from the University of California, Irvine, and a master's degree in sacred music and cantorial investiture from Hebrew Union College–Jewish Insitute of Religion. Lisa's original musical compositions have appeared in dozens of publications and recordings and are sung in congregations around the world. She has released two songbooks and six CDs, including *Mis Canciones Para Los Judios de Cuba* ("My Songs for the Jews of Cuba"), which features the music she performed in two concerts in Havana in 2006 and 2007. Lisa is an active member of the Washington, DC–area Jewish community with her husband, Andy, and their two teenage children.

CAROL KRUCOFF, E-RYT, is a yoga therapist at Duke Integrative Medicine in Durham, North Carolina. An award-winning journalist and fitness expert, Carol served as founding editor of the health section of the *Washington Post*, where her syndicated column, "Bodyworks," appeared for twelve years. Carol is the author of *Healing Yoga for Neck and Shoulder Pain*, co-author with husband Mitchell Krucoff, MD, of *Healing Moves: How to Cure, Relieve and Prevent Common Ailments with Exercise*, and creator of the home practice CD *Healing Moves Yoga*. A frequent contributor to *Yoga Journal*, she has written for numerous national publications including the *New York Times*, the *Huffington Post*, *Prevention*, and *Reader's Digest*. Carol is a member of Judea Reform Congregation in Durham, North Carolina, and is active in the larger Chapel Hill-Durham Jewish community with her husband and their two adult children.